A History

of Art Therapy

in the United States

Maxine Borowsky Junge
with Paige Pateracki Asawa

Published by The American Art Therapy Association, Inc.

Please write to:
The American Art Therapy Association, Inc.
1202 Allanson Road
Mundelein, Illinois 60060
708/949-6064

ISBN 1-882-147-23-5 (paperback)

445

Book & Cover Design
Paige Pateracki Asawa

 Printed on recycled paper

To my first teachers who, through their lives, showed me how to integrate the arts and therapy—Eula Long, art teacher, Ruth Adams, cello teacher, and my father Marvin Borowsky, writer, painter, and teacher. And to Helen Landgarten who involved me in the formal business of art therapy, nurtured me, and made certain I stayed.

With love,

M.B.J

*C*ontents

We thank those publishers and/or copyright holders who have given permission for excerpts from the following books and articles to be reprinted in this work:

Gladys Agell, Editor of the *American Journal of Art Therapy,* and Vermont College of Norwich University, Northfield, VT
  An interview with Edith Kramer, J. McMahan, *American Journal of Art Therapy, 27,* 4, 1989
  An interview with Elinor Ulman, H. Jordan, *American Journal of Art Therapy, 26, 4,* 1988
Brunner/Mazel, New York, NY
  Approaches to Art Therapy, Judith Rubin (Editor), 1987
  The Art of Art Therapy, Judith Rubin, 1984
  Family Art Psychotherapy, Helen B. Landgarten, 1987
Human Sciences Press, New York, NY
  The Artist as Therapist, Arthur Robbins, 1987
  The Psychoaesthetic Experience, Arthur Robbins, 1989
Claire Levy, Art Therapy Publications, Craftsbury Commons, VT
  The Artist in Each of Us, Florence Cane, 1983
  Roots of art therapy: Margaret Naumburg (1890-1983) and Florence Cane (1882-1952) - A family portrait. *American Journal of Art Therapy, 22, 4,* 1983
  Meaning in art therapy. *Bulletin of Art Therapy, 2, 2,* 1962
  Art Therapy in Theory and Practice, Elinor Ulman & Penny Dachinger, Eds. Schoken Books, New York, NY
Magnolia Street Publishers, Chicago, IL
  The Gestalt Art Experience, Janie Rhyne, 1984
  Dynamically Oriented Art Therapy: Its Principles and Practice, Margaret Naumburg, 1987
Schocken Books, New York, NY
  Art as Therapy with Children, Edith Kramer, 1971
Charles C Thomas, Publisher, Springfield, IL
  Art Therapy in a Children's Community, Edith Kramer, 1958
  Educating the Creative Arts Therapist: A Profile of the Profession, Shaun McNiff, 1986
  Family Therapy and Evaluation through Art, Hanna Yaxa Kwiatkowska, 1978
  Self-Discovery through Self-Expression, Mala Betensky, 1973
  The Arts and Psychotherapy, Shaun McNiff, 1981
  The Psychocybernetic Model of Art Therapy, Aina O. Nucho, 1987
  They Could not Talk and So They Drew: Children's Styles of Coping and Thinking, Myra Levick, 1983
John Wiley & Sons, New York, NY

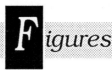igures

*F*oreword

What could be a more fitting way to commemorate the 25th anniversary of the American Art Therapy Association than to publish a monograph documenting the history of the profession of art therapy and the development of AATA? Individual historic accounts and remembrances have proliferated over the past 25 years, but these scattered reports have made it all but impossible to understand and appreciate our roots.

Maxine Borowsky Junge, Ph.D., A.T.R., has spent nine years gathering these and other diverse pieces of memories, recollections, and material from or about many of the pioneers who founded our profession. The American Art Therapy Association is pleased to present the results of her efforts—*A History of Art Therapy in the United States.*

This text, well researched and written by Dr. Junge with the assistance of Paige Pateracki Asawa, is a study of the foundations of the profession of art therapy and the development of the American Art Therapy Association. It is with great pride that AATA publishes it to benefit students, mental health professionals, members of AATA, and supporters of the field. We commend Dr. Junge for her scholarly efforts and insights and for providing a text that will surely inspire other art therapists to research, remember, and record the missing pieces of our past.

We congratulate Dr. Junge and Ms. Asawa on their efforts and their timely completion of this informative and valuable resource. And we thank them for a most fitting and appropriate 25th anniversary present.

Bobbi Stoll, M.F.C.C., L.A.T., A.T.R.
President, 1993–1995
The American Art Therapy Association

Acknowledgments

Linda Gantt has played a major role in helping this history see daylight and I owe her a huge debt of thanks. I am grateful for her respect and appreciation for the work, her encyclopaedic knowledge of the field, and her precise attention to detail. Linda's even spirit and emotional support have aided immeasurably, and in the last stages, her warm home in the snowy woods of West Virginia sustained me.

Many art therapists contributed information to this project. Some of them are Bernard Stone, Cay Drachnik, Linda Gantt, Judy Rubin, and Helen Landgarten. The American Art Therapy Association Archives at the Menninger Foundation in Topeka, Kansas were made available as was the Mary Huntoon Collection at the University of Kansas. During my hours in the dust and stacks, Bob and Marilyn Ault supported me with hospitality.

Paige Pateracki Asawa signed onto the project relatively late, but has been invaluable; her research and computer skills have considerably enriched the manuscript. I am indebted to Paige and the other art therapy students Joan Bosky, Noah Hass-Cohen, Rosalyn Kleiman, Jasenka Roje, and Robin Spector, who allowed me to use some of their work in the literature section.

The history originated during my doctoral work at the Fielding Institute and I thank Jody Veroff and Anna DiStefano for their interest and reading of the first manuscript.

Finally, I thank Patricia Allen, the AATA Publications Chair who first suggested that this history be published by the American Art Therapy Association, and Cathy Malchiodi who as a member of AATA's Board of Directors helped keep the project alive.

Many quotations in the text contain the sexist language typical of the time and culture. This language has been retained in the interests of historical accuracy and flavor.

Maxine Borowsky Junge,
Ph.D., L.C.S.W., A.T.R.
Los Angeles, California
September, 1994

Without a doubt, my first thanks must go to Maxine Junge for inviting me to participate in this most important undertaking. I deeply appreciate the opportunity to contribute to the writing of the history and to forge and strengthen our friendship in the process.

My thanks also go to Linda Gantt for her unending support, no matter what the obstacle. Her determination and attention to detail have proved invaluable in taking the manuscript the final yards.

Finally, I thank my family who have contributed from the distant past and the present in ways that words can not express. I would especially like to thank my perennially patient husband who graciously gave many hours of at-home time on the computer (when we had only one) and support throughout the stages of the work.

Paige Pateracki Asawa, M.A.
Los Angeles, California
September, 1994

I ntroduction

When I (MBJ) was twelve years old, I attended a children's Saturday art class at the Kann Institute of Art in Los Angeles. The teacher, an energetic gray-haired woman named Eula Long, was interested in the psychological aspects of the creative process and, in particular, was a student of Gestalt psychology which she used to inform her teaching with the normal and troubled children in her classes. She believed that a supportive emotional environment was essential to the creation of art— that no child's art should be criticized but only praised, and that the teaching of technique was not only unimportant but hindered or even stopped the child's creativity entirely. She discouraged the visual clichés and stereotypes that typically represent a defensiveness against an inner process of exploration and she valued fantasy, imagination, and the directness of feeling essential to all true artistic products. I attended Eula's classes until I was fifteen and began "real" art school with adults on Saturdays, in addition to my high school work. There, I found that mostly technical skills were taught and the inner spirit of art, the creative process itself was seldom encouraged or nurtured.

Those three years of classes were not called art therapy and Eula Long did not refer to herself as an art therapist but I am convinced that that was what she was. I watched my drawings and paintings, at first stilted and self-conscious, take on a richness and excitement that began to be recognized by parents, teachers, and friends. With Eula, I had the privilege of experiencing the therapeutic power and the possibility intrinsic in art. My life was irrevocably changed and Eula Long, in large measure, contributed to my later career as an art therapist.

Years later, in 1974, when I serendipitously stumbled into the profession of art therapy and had found a way to put art, creativity, and my interest in working with people together, I began to teach in the new graduate program in art therapy, initiated by Helen Landgarten at Immaculate Heart College in Los Angeles. There, I looked for some kind of written history of the field to present to my students and found none that seemed to represent the scope and depth of the field that even I, as a novice, had discovered. I knew I was engaged in a new and innovative profession, but I also was aware that art therapy had been defined as a separate discipline since the 1940s. Apparently, like my art teacher Eula Long, the talented clinicians who were art therapy's pioneers were too busy creating history to write about it. Although some art therapy books had been published, I found them generally disappointing in terms of their presentation of history. Many authors tried to define the field, its present reality and potential, but what little attention was paid to history tended to focus on the writer's own particular experience and geographical area. Since the early writers came from the New York and Washington, DC, areas, and the journal (*The Bulletin of Art Therapy*), came out of Washington, it appeared to me that art therapy had not only its origins but its continuing major existence on the East Coast. I knew this not to be the whole story by any means. In 1977, a definitive chapter entitled "Art Therapy" appeared in the book *Interdisciplinary Approaches to Human Services* (Valletutti and Christoplos, 1977). This chapter was reprinted as a monograph in 1978 under the title of *Art Therapy in the United States*. The authors were Elinor Ulman, Edith Kramer, and Hanna Yaxa Kwiatkowska, three well–respected authors and clinicians (Ms. Ulman had founded and edited the *Bulletin*) from the East Coast "bloc." Covering a broad variety of issues in the field, the monograph's historical survey remained narrowly focused primarily on its three authors with the addition of the Gestalt art therapist Janie Rhyne. More recent writings have tended to perpetuate this view.

All written history is determined by the perceptions, attitudes, and choices of those who write it and who thereby determine our views, but I must admit this persistence of geographical limitation rankled me. I had been an art therapist, clinician, and teacher for some time and had found art therapy to be a field of immense vitality, scope, and variety. I had also met art therapists from across the country, many of whom had been practicing for years and had been actively involved in the formulation and expansion of art therapy as a mental health discipline and as a profession. Why were their names and accomplishments not listed among the others? Finally in 1981, a chapter titled "Art Therapy: An Overview" by Myra Levick appeared in the *Handbook of Innovative Psychotherapies* (Corsini, 1981). Levick's history included a broader selection of art therapists and a more extensive geographical range. For example, mentioned for the first time was the active group in Kansas which had been connected to the Menninger Foundation since the early 1950s. At last, someone was on the right track, I thought.

One of my (PPA) first classes in the graduate art therapy program at Loyola Marymount, was Art Therapy

Literature. I remember feeling very excited, having already read some of the literature, to dive into the wealth of material written on the field of art therapy. To my dismay the field lacked any sort of written comprehensive history. There were articles here and there and introductory chapters in books but no published history. It seemed unbelievable that this could be the case in a field that has been in existence since the 1940s.

It was in this same literature class that I was first given a copy of Maxine's initial work on this history. I was satisfied that at least someone was concerned about this obvious gap in the literature. Not only did the absence of a published history affect students of art therapy but also those from other disciplines who had a general interest in the field but could not find out about its development from a single source. Needless to say, I became actively interested in the project upon which Maxine had embarked and helped form a student group to investigate the various theorists whose work is described in Chapter 4. The entire group worked hard to grasp the core meaning of the various views so that we could begin to gain perspective on the field and develop our own individual styles of art therapy.

Through the process of writing about the authors of the first and second generations I came to realize how these pioneers set the stage for the development of the field. They forged a foundation with their strong will and determination. It seems imperative for students and professionals alike to gain an awareness of these underpinnings in order to understand the spirit of art therapy in general and the American Art Therapy Association specifically.

When Maxine invited me to work on the history I was ecstatic. What an important mission—to help get the history out into the world. I thought of all the future generations of students who would not have to wonder, as I did, why there was no published history. I also thought of what a wonderful tool this will be for other mental health professionals who are interested in our field.

The American Art Therapy Association has developed guidelines for Master's degree academic programs for the training of art therapists. The guidelines require that the history of art therapy be studied and that "emphasis should be placed on the extensive history of the discipline including reference to the works of early and contemporary practitioners" (American Art Therapy Association, *Guidelines for Academic, Institute, and Clinical Art Therapy Training,* January 1, 1993, p. 4). Since the literature to date has not, in my (MBJ) judgment, adequately addressed this injunction, and because of my own needs in teaching, I decided to undertake the task of putting together a more encompassing history of art therapy in the hope that it will be a contribution to the field and to the students now and to come.

This monograph is our attempt to broaden the base for study and to highlight some of the many dedicated women and men who have contributed in so many ways. Clearly, this cannot be a comprehensive history. There will be inevitable omissions since, like those writers before us, we too are limited in information and have made particular choices. Fortunately, because art therapy is a relatively new endeavor, much is still "living history" and there are those who can tell us what is missing.

Sources for this history are the books and papers written by art therapists over the last twenty-five years; the set of oral histories of art therapy pioneers (a project of the University of Louisville in 1975); documents from the archives of the American Art Therapy Association, kept at the Menninger Foundation in Topeka, Kansas; the Mary Huntoon collection at the University of Kansas in Lawrence; and the personal communications of many art therapists across the country for which we are very grateful. My (MBJ) colleague Helen Landgarten, a pioneer art therapist and a member of the first Executive

Board of the American Art Therapy Association, suggested this project and opened her extensive files to me. Without her help, this monograph would not have been possible.

We have organized this information into five chapters: Precursors and Influences; The Formative Years; Expansion and Consolidation; The Art Therapy Literature; and Building on the Past. In each chapter we have tried to point out what we judge to be important trends and developments as well as art therapy's relationship with its context: psychoanalysis, psychiatry, and the mental health disciplines on the one hand, and art education on the other. We have also tried to underscore those ongoing issues that have at once enlivened, and at times, frustrated art therapy's evolution. A chronology is included.

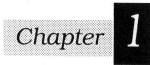

Chapter 1

Precursors

&

Influences

Art therapy's roots extend as far back as prehistory when people drew images in caves in an attempt to express and master their world. An early example of the specific use of the arts in healing is found in biblical sources which discuss David's attempt to cure King Saul's depression by playing the harp for him (I Samuel 16, verses 14–23). From Navaho sandpaintings to African sculpture, many examples can be found of the use of visual arts in therapeutic ritual.

The development of art therapy as a profession is usually dated from the 1940s, the decade in which Margaret Naumburg began publishing her work. However, a number of intellectual and sociological developments in the late 19th and early 20th centuries gave rise to the climate in which Naumburg's ideas took hold. More humane treatment of mental patients, the child study movement, anthropological expeditions to non-Western cultures, the development of psychotropic drugs, progressive education, new theories in philosophy and psychology, and the refining of the scientific method, all would have a significant effect on the development of art therapy theory and practice.

INFLUENCES FROM PSYCHOLOGY & PSYCHIATRY

Personality Theories

Art therapy evolved directly out of the personality theories of Freud, Jung, and others and, in particular, from the theory and techniques of psychoanalysis. Freud's powerful concept of the unconscious and the idea that memories, thoughts, and feelings are expressed symbolically in our dreams provided an important theoretical base for art therapy. Freud stated:

> We experience it [a dream] predominantly in visual images; feelings may be present too, and thoughts interwoven in it as well; the other senses may also experience something, but nonetheless it is predominantly a question

of images. Part of the difficulty of giving an account of dreams is due to our having to translate these images into words. "I could draw it," a dreamer often says to us, "but I don't know how to say it." (Freud, 1963, p. 90)

Jung's formulation of a collective unconscious with a cross-cultural symbolism passed on through generations has had a particular impact on art therapy as well. Jung's interest in the psychological meanings inherent in artwork, especially the *mandala* ("magic circle" in Sanskrit) (Jung, 1972), and his fascination with his own drawings and those of his patients were also influential. Unlike Freud, who never asked his patients to draw the imagery of their dreams, Jung often urged his patients to do so. "To paint what we see before us," Jung wrote, "is a different art from painting what we see within" (Jung, 1954, p. 253). Michael Edwards, a British art therapist points out:

Freud had, of course, led the way in giving recognition and importance to such imagery, especially in dreams, but there is an important distinction to be made. Freud treated the dream, the fantasy, or the unconscious factor in a picture as a puzzle to be solved and explained in terms of psychoanalytic theory, whereas Jung attempted to relate to the unconscious image as an entity in its own right. In doing so he examined images from a number of perspectives, cultural as well as psychological. It is an open, hermeneutic mode of interpretation, lacking the economy and elegance of Freud's method, but offering instead a psychological reevaluation of traditional ways of understanding inner experience. (Edwards, 1987, pp. 93–94)

Art from Untrained Artists

A primary factor in the eventual evolution of art therapy was the accumulation of scholarly books and articles on the artwork of the insane as well as that of children and non-Western cultures. European psychiatrists such as Lombroso, Tardieu, and Simon were writing about their patients' art over a hundred years ago (MacGregor, 1983). There are several detailed surveys and bibliographies of the early literature on psychiatric art including those by MacGregor (1989), Kiell (1965), and Anastasi and Foley (1940, 1941a, & 1941b). Harris (1963) provides a thorough historical review of the earliest studies of children's drawings.

At the beginning of the 20th century, the European psychiatrists Kraepelin, Jaspers, and Aschaffenburg "came to the conclusion that the drawings of psychotics were an as yet undeveloped source of psychiatric knowledge which was especially useful as an aid in diagnosis" (Naumburg, 1950, p. 10). Some in the European psychiatric community considered the drawings and paintings by patients in psychiatric hospitals as having aesthetic value as works of art. A Heidelberg art historian and psychiatrist Hans Prinzhorn collected more than 5,000 pieces of artwork (MacGregor, 1989, p. 194) produced by patients in psychiatric hospitals and published a book on his collection in 1922, *Artistry of the Mentally Ill*. (This work was later translated into English; see Prinzhorn, 1972).

Prinzhorn was interested primarily in the remarkable and sometimes bizarre aesthetic quality of the art of mental patients. His aim was to identify the aspects common to all art making regardless of the mental condition of the person who made it. He did not consider, however, that the creative process might possibly be therapeutic for the patient or an aid to the diagnosis of psychopathology.

In another European publication, *Insania Pingens* (Cocteau, Schmidt, Steck, & Bader, 1961), which has an introduction by artist and filmmaker Jean Cocteau, two psychiatrists, both directors of psychiatric hospitals, and a professor at the Academy of Plastic Arts in Munich presented visually compelling art by psychotic patients along with a discussion about its aesthetic value. Although no therapeutic role for the art was indicated, Dr. Alfred Bader, in his section titled "The Pictorial Work of

Psychotics—A Mirror of the Human Soul," suggests the reflective and diagnostic potential of a patient's art.

Psychological Tests

The psychological techniques known as projective tests are closely related to assessment through art. Leonardo da Vinci may have given us a first example of a projective test when he reported in his *Introduction to the Painter* about the associative possibilities raised when viewing a blot made by throwing a sponge upon a wall:

> various experiences can be seen in such a blot, provided one wants to find them in it—human heads, various animals, battles, cliffs, seas, clouds or forests and other things. (Leonardo da Vinci quoted in Zubin, Eron, & Shumer, 1965, p. 167)

Psychologists interested in measuring quantitative information about the personality have experimented with the use of visual stimuli and inkblots to elicit associative responses. The Rorschach Test, first published in Europe in 1921 and imported to this country around 1925, provided ambiguous inkblots to evoke emotional and associative responses. The Thematic Apperception Test (TAT), published in 1938, used imaginative productions such as stories told in response to a series of pictures.[1]

Since the 1940s, an individual's drawings have generally been assumed to be a visual representation of an internal state, although the research evidence to support this remains contradictory. In 1926, Florence Goodenough designed an intelligence test for children based primarily on the number of details included in the drawing of a man. She and other clinicians became aware that the "Draw-A-Man" test seemed to be tapping into personality characteristics in addition to intellectual capabilities. John Buck's "House-Tree-Person" procedure (1948) and Karen Machover's "Draw-A-Person" technique (Machover, 1949) developed as a result of their experiences with intelligence tests. These standardized drawing tests were based on the postulate that projective drawings could be used as a clinical tool through which a person's inner world may be seen and understood.

INFLUENCES FROM EDUCATION

Progressive Education

In the late 19th century, psychologists and educators began to apply scientific methods to the study of childhood. The results of their observations were then integrated into various theories which were, in turn, applied to educational programs. Realizing that children went through specific stages of development, writers such as

Jean Piaget, Maria Montessori, and John Dewey advocated tailoring schools to individual needs rather than relying on rote memorization and inculcation. The progressive education movement which began at the end of the 19th century was

> a reaction to the alleged narrowness and formalism of traditional education. One of its main objectives was to educate the "whole child".... Creative and manual arts gained importance in the curriculum, and children were encouraged toward experimentation and independent thinking. (*Encyclopaedia Britannica*, 1980, VIII, p. 232)

The interest in developmental stages then led to research in what seemed to be the predictable development of children's drawing abilities, and the emphasis on the creative arts gave rise to new teaching techniques.

Modern Art Education

The work of the pioneers of modern art education such as Franz Cizek, Viktor Lowenfeld, and Florence Cane were especially influential in the development of art therapy. Cizek, a Viennese, was interested in the natural development of children's artistic abilities and stressed the importance of the free expression of imagination and creativity in artwork. Cizek also served as a mentor for

Viktor Lowenfeld, one of the most widely read art educators in this country. Lowenfeld studied psychoanalysis in Vienna before coming to the United States. *Creative and Mental Growth*, Lowenfeld's classic book, first published in 1947, proposed the idea that a child's intellectual growth is connected to creative development and, therefore, that art is essential in all education:

> The process of drawing, painting, or constructing is a complex one in which the child brings together diverse elements of his environment to make a new meaningful whole. In the process of selecting, interpreting and reforming these elements, he has given us more than a picture, he has given us a part of himself...for the child this is a dynamic and unifying activity. (Lowenfeld, 1964, p. 1)

Furthermore, Lowenfeld described a predictable sequence[2] in the development of a child's art and demonstrated evidence for a stage theory of growth. According to Lowenfeld, a child progresses through six typical stages. Beginning with the "Scribbling Stage" (ages 2 to 4), the child moves to the "Preschematic Stage" (4 to 7) in which the first attempts at representing the world are made, then to the "Schematic Stage" (7 to 9), the "Gang Age" (9 to 11), the "Pseudo-Naturalistic Stage" (11 to 13) and the "Period of Decision: The Crisis of Adolescence." He also worked with physically and mentally handicapped children, using artwork to enhance a sense of identity.[3]

THE NAUMBURG SISTERS & THE WALDEN SCHOOL

It was from this matrix of new educational and psychological theories, mixed with the influence of Cubist and Surrealist art, that the Naumburg sisters began to build a scaffold of ideas about the therapeutic use of art.

⌈While most art therapists acknowledge Margaret Naumburg as the mother of art therapy, relatively few realize the part that her older sister Florence Cane played in the field's eventual development. From these two extraordinary women came the foundation for what would be eventually considered as the two ends of the art therapy spectrum.⌉

> Florence Cane was an artist and art teacher; Margaret Naumburg, an educator who became a psychologist and art therapist.... Fundamentally their work does not conflict but is complementary. Florence developed teaching methods to free artistic expression; building on Florence's achievement, Margaret concentrated on developing methods of therapy using art. (Kniazzeh in Detre et al., 1983, pp. 111–112)

Margaret Naumburg

Born in 1882, Margaret Naumburg had a successful career as an innovator in education before she turned to art therapy well past middle age. Naumburg was educated at Vassar and Barnard Colleges and did graduate work at Columbia University with John Dewey and at the London School of Economics with Beatrice and Sidney Webb. She also studied in Italy with Maria Montessori. According to her son, Thomas Frank:

> Long before I appeared on the scene, Margaret Naumburg and her husband the author Waldo Frank, were part of a literary-artistic circle in New York City that included the photographer Alfred Stieglitz, the poet Hart Crane, painters such as John Marin, Georgia O'Keeffe, and Marsden Hartley, and from the West Coast film industry, Charlie Chaplin. As well, the European painters Matisse, Braque, and Picasso were first exhibited in this country by Stieglitz at his gallery, An American Place. There among this circle of vigorous contributors to all the arts, Margaret Naumburg's interest in symbolism and primitive art must have been stirred. During those same early years, she was beginning to participate actively in the progressive education movement. (Frank in Detre et al., 1983, pp. 112–113)

In 1915,[4] Naumburg founded the Walden School (originally called the Children's School) in New York

City, a progressive school "established on the basic psychoanalytic insights concerning the importance of the unconscious in education as well as in psychotherapy" (Naumburg, 1966, p. 30). At Walden, Naumburg put into practice her conviction that the emotional development of children, fostered through encouragement of spontaneous creative expression and self-motivated learning, should take precedence over the traditional intellectual approach to the teaching of a standardized curriculum (Frank in Detre et al., 1983, p. 113).

Naumburg's son quotes from an essay his mother wrote which was found among her papers. Across the top of the paper titled "A Direct Method of Education," she had scrawled "First application of psychoanalysis to education in the U.S. 1917" (p. 113). In her essay Naumburg wrote:

> Up to the present, our methods of education have dealt only with the conscious or surface mental life of the child. The new analytic psychology has, however, demonstrated that the unconscious mental life which is the outgrowth of the child's instincts plays a greater role than the conscious.... The new psychology has uncovered the true nature of primitive thought and has shown that it still lives on in the unconscious mental being of the adult as well as of the child....

> This discovery of the fundamental sources of thought and action must now bring about a readjustment in education. (Naumburg quoted by Frank in Detre et al., 1983, p. 113)

This relationship of psychoanalytic theory and education flourished as "a number of artists, writers, and professors, as well as some well-known psychoanalysts (such as Dr. A. A. Brill and Dr. Leonard Blumgart), sent their children to Walden" (Naumburg, 1966, p. 30). With Naumburg's encouragement, many teachers undertook personal analyses. Naumburg herself underwent an analysis with a Jungian, Dr. Beatrice Hinkle, and later, a second analysis with Dr. Brill, the premier American Freudian.

It is interesting that the break between Jung and Freud happened after the 1912 publication of Jung's *Wandlungen und Symbole der Libido* which presented a theory about symbolism quite different from Freud. This work was first translated to English in 1916 as *Psychology of the Unconscious* by Naumburg's analyst Beatrice Hinkle. Both Naumburg and her sister Florence Cane underwent analysis with Hinkle indicating a decided Jungian attraction and influence. Naumburg's inner circle of friends was highly educated and many underto Freudian analysis themselves. Naumburg seems to ha staked out a neutral theoretical ground for herself in declaring that "such conflicting interpretations [Freudian and Jungian] point to the need of giving further attention to encouraging patients to make more interpretations of their own symbolic material. For it is on the basis of each patient's response to his own symbolic creations that the importance of using spontaneous art projections as a primary mode of therapy can be established" (Naumburg, 1950, pp. 33–34).

Along with being Director of Walden, Naumburg taught art to the children of the school. She came to believe in art as a form of "symbolic speech basic to all education" and grew convinced that "such spontaneous art expression was also basic to psychotherapeutic treatment" (Naumburg, 1966, p. 30). Dismayed by the usual education for teachers, Naumburg employed people who lacked traditional training but were exciting individuals, some of whom would make significant contributions of their own to arts and letters; Lewis Mumford taught English, Hendrik van Loon taught history, and Ernest Bloch taught music (Frank in Detre et al., 1983, p. 113).

Florence Cane

Naumburg's sister Florence Cane, a gifted art teacher, was deeply influenced by psychoanalytic thinking and underwent a Jungian analysis. At a time when most teaching of art meant instruction in skills toward realistic rendering as the goal, Cane realized the importance of the emotions as a source for creativity. Florence Cane, came to teach art at Walden about 1920. According to one of her daughters, Cane criticized the art teaching because "creativity and individuality were being crushed," and "begged Margaret to let her experiment with one class" (Robinson, 1983, p. ii). In addition, Cane worked as Director of Art for the Counseling Centre for Gifted Children of the School of Education of New York University for 14 years (Detre et al., 1983, p. 117), had her own school, and took students referred to her by analysts.

Cane developed methods to help free the child from defensive stereotypic drawing and painting. These included, among others, the use of movement, sound, and the scribble technique, and had as their goal loosening defenses, evoking a type of free association, and tapping into fantasies and the unconscious. Cane's daughter Mary Cane Robinson remembers her mother as a teacher:

Winnicott
"scribble technique"

> I recall a picture I made in the mid-1920s when Florence was teaching at the Walden School and I was a 16-year-old student in her class. It was called "Despair." Each member of the class was to choose a mood or feeling; we were to

act it out through movement and gesture; make sketches of it; find the colors and environmental forms or shapes to express this feeling; then organize all this into a painting. I can just see us moving, dancing, what-you-will, to express Struggle, Pain, and Joy. The class was alive, deeply engaged. Why do I recall that particular painting? It was a *whole* experience, using the three functions—movement, feeling, thought—espoused in Florence's theory to integrate the person with the product. (Robinson in Detre et al., 1983, p. 117)

Florence Cane's book *The Artist in Each of Us* was first published in 1951. She died in 1952, leaving art education and art therapy an important legacy. Many of her ideas and methods concerning the release of unconscious imagery are still viewed as controversial in art education. Cane wrote:

this awakening [of the spirit cannot] be won in the method adopted by some moderns.... But this is ... a middle path where ... the teacher's role becomes that of a lover and student of human beings, whose aim is to release the essential nature of the child and to let that nature create its own form of expression, beginning in play and growing into effort. The integrity of the child is preserved and the art produced is genuine, primitive, and true. (Cane, 1929, p. 125)

Many art therapists today may be unaware that some psychiatrists referred patients to Cane. In a brief passage, she mentions how she worked with such cases:

> ...drawing from the unconscious is definitely used for the purpose of healing. This collaboration with the analyst is possible because my work does not cut across the patient's transference to the analyst. I function as the creative teacher, perceiving the meaning of the pupil's work, but leaving the analysis to the psychiatrist. (Cane, 1983, p. 10)

Here she succinctly describes the stance she took on interpretation of the art, a stance which clearly set her apart from Naumburg. Cane states that there are

> many instances when the patient or student requires medical care, but...a great deal of healing can take place through the catharsis of art under the guidance of a teacher who understands the meanings shown in the paintings and the unexpressed needs of the child and who possesses the ability to help the child cleanse and renew himself. (p. 10)

Although "art therapy is not identical with art teaching, progressive art teaching methods are indispensable tools in therapeutic art programs" (Kramer, 1971b, p. 8). Florence Cane's book, long out of print, has been republished (Cane, 1983), making her exciting work accessible to new generations of artists, art educators, and art therapists.

In the space of less than 5 years the Naumburg sisters had published three books (Naumburg, 1947, 1950; Cane, 1951) which would define what later became the two poles of the field of art therapy in the 1960s and 1970s. But they were not the only ones who were discovering the potent combination of art and therapy. The intellectual climate provided a fertile mix of new ideas in psychological and educational theories, treatment techniques, and developments in modern art, philosophy, and the social sciences. Many artists who had never heard of Naumburg or Cane responded to this *Zeitgeist* and began working, often as volunteers, in a variety of therapeutic and rehabilitative programs, thinking that they had invented a field which would be called art therapy.

Notes:

[1] See Groth-Marnat (1990) for a detailed history and discussion of the Rorschach, the TAT, and projective drawings.

2 Lowenfeld's idea of predictable "stages" in children's art was not entirely innovative since Cooke had published an article on the subject in 1885, and Kerschensteiner classified drawings according to three main stages in his book published in 1905 (Gantt, 1991, personal communication).

3 The chapter "Therapeutic Aspects of Art Education" in the third edition of Lowenfeld's *Creative and Mental Growth* (1957) which dealt with this aspect of his work was dropped from later editions. That excised material was republished in the *American Journal of Art Therapy*, Volume 25, Number 4, 1987.

4 Some sources such as Detre et al. (1983) cite 1914 as the date of the founding of the school. Perhaps the discrepancy stems from the name change.

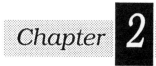

Chapter 2

The
Formative Years

In the United States, art therapy comes primarily out of the psychoanalytic tradition. With the expanding interest in and knowledge of psychoanalysis, a few artists and art educators combined their skill in art with the study of analytic theory, sometimes undergoing personal analyses. This synergy between art and psychology eventually came to be called art therapy. Others, such as Ainslie Meares (1957, 1958, 1960), an Australian psychiatrist, and M. A. Sechehaye (1951), a Swiss psychoanalyst, saw the importance of accepting and understanding the personal symbols of severely regressed patients. Reviewing their books, Elinor Ulman writes:

The Door of Serenity by Ainslie Meares is a psychiatric story of the intensive treatment of a patient whose expressive powers were so terribly impoverished that for a long time painting was the only communication she could attempt. With no direct guidance, she progressed from depicting her symptoms to revealing the conflicts underlying them, and finally to expressing the largely unconscious symbolism of those conflicts. [This work] invites comparison with M. A. Sechehaye's *Symbolic Realization*, published some years before. (Ulman, 1960, p. 113)

MARGARET NAUMBURG: THE MOTHER OF ART THERAPY

Although others had called themselves art therapists and had written about their work prior to 1940,[1] Margaret Naumburg was the first to delineate art therapy as a separate profession and a distinct form of psychotherapy. Her integration of ideas from a variety of sources into a coherent system of principles formed a persuasive paradigm. Through her books, articles, lectures, courses, and exhibits at professional conferences, her contribution was immense.[2]

Art therapy has sometimes been called "a technique in search of a theory" (Rubin, 1978, p. 18). Naumburg's work which she called "Dynamically Oriented Art Therapy" adopted Freud's dictum that the unconscious speaks in imagery, and she asked her patients to draw those images. Naumburg said "Art therapy recognizes that the unconscious as expressed in a patient's phantasies, daydreams and fears can be projected more immediately in pictures than in words" (Naumburg, 1966, p. 3). Naumburg integrated the theory and techniques of psychoanalysis with her own theory and methods for using drawing and personal symbolism in therapy.

After leaving the directorship of Walden School in the early 1920s, Naumburg bore her son Thomas, divorced her husband Waldo Frank, and lived in the West for a few years.[3] In addition, she wrote a book on education and her experience at Walden called *The Child and the World* (1928). Eventually, she met Nolan D. C. Lewis, Director of the New York State Psychiatric Institute who for many years had used free paintings in therapy with his adult patients (Lewis, 1925, 1928). Naumburg credits Lewis as being "the first psychiatrist to employ analysis of the art productions of patients either singly or in series, as an adjunct to psychoanalytic treatment" (Naumburg, 1950, p. 13). Naumburg writes:

> I asked [Lewis] whether he might be interested in an experimental research program in the use of spontaneous art in therapy with some of the behavior-problem children in

his hospital. His immediate and sympathetic response to this idea was based on his own experience as to the value of spontaneous art with his own patients. (Naumburg, 1966, p. 30)

Naumburg's research at the New York State Institute covered 6 years (1941 to 1947) and extended from dynamically oriented art therapy with children to the use of spontaneous art with adults diagnosed with schizophrenia. She published this work in 1947 as a book with the lengthy title of *Studies of the "Free" Expression of Behavior Problem Children as a Means of Diagnosis and Therapy.*[4] In this book and later ones, Naumburg suggested that dynamically oriented art therapy is based on:

the recognition that man's fundamental thoughts and feelings are derived from the unconscious and often reach expression in images rather than in words. By means of pictorial projection, art therapy encourages a method of symbolic communication between patient and therapist. (Naumburg, 1966, p. 1)

Naumburg proposed that once patients had created nonverbal spontaneous imagery they would make verbal associations to their pictures. Convinced that art was a more direct route than words to the unconscious, she found that the use of expressive art could speed up the therapeutic process:

Art therapy...encourages...an expression of inner experience. Objectified picturization acts then as an immediate symbolic communication which frequently circumvents the difficulties of speech. Another advantage inherent in the making of unconscious pictured projections is that such symbolic images more easily escape repression by what Freud called the mind's "censor" than do verbal expressions, which are more familiar to the patient. (p. 2)

Naumburg believed that art therapy, like psychoanalysis, takes place within a transference relationship, but she departed from traditional analytic techniques in that she insisted that the patient sit upright, take an active rather than a dependent role, and analyze and interpret his or her own imagery:

diff w/ Sista

Thus a patient is gradually assisted to recognize that his artistic productions can be treated as a mirror in which he can begin to find his own motives revealed....

The patient is gradually freed from overdependence on the therapist who withholds interpretation and thereby encourages the patient to discover for himself what his symbolic pictures mean to him. (p. 3)

Margaret Naumburg's formulation clearly focused on the *therapy* part rather than the *art* aspect. Naumburg did not stress the creation of an aesthetic product. She believed that spontaneous art, even of those who were untrained, could be valuable in releasing and projecting unconscious conflicts and providing symbolic communication between patient and therapist. Critics of Naumburg's theory have suggested that for her, art becomes merely an additional tool for verbal psychotherapy.

In her de-emphasis of the art product and her focus on the integration of art and psychotherapy, Naumburg articulated what would become one perspective of an ongoing and heated debate among art therapists that continues to this day. Although she had conducted art classes at Walden, Naumburg's psychotherapy emphasis conflicted with the beliefs of some other art therapists who had been or were art educators and who placed the greatest importance on the creation of art and contended that the locus of therapy was within the creative process itself. A theory which centered on the art-making aspect of art therapy would not be formally articulated until much later by Edith Kramer.

Margaret Naumburg died in her sleep February 26, 1983, at the age of 93.[5] Her son remembers her years as a fighter for her new insights:

> I have clear memories of my mother as a fighter against the establishment, against the inevitable resistance to new ideas and concepts. Earlier she had battled for her experi-

mental school, which went counter to traditional approaches in education by championing the child's freedom of emotional expression....I recall hearing her tell often how she had to fight established psychiatry's opposition to her research with patients. She was forever pointing out that art therapy, with its use of symbolic language and imagery was often a more effective road to the unconscious than the usual verbal approach of psychoanalysis and dynamic psychotherapy. (Frank in Detre et al., 1983, p. 114)

After her death, Rudolf Arnheim, author and Professor Emeritus of the Psychology of Art at Harvard University, assessed Naumburg's contribution:

Perhaps it is in the nature of a new discipline that it starts with a great figure of a founder whom nobody in particular has taught the things he or she will teach the first generation of regular professionals. (Arnheim, 1984, p. 3)

Arnheim highlighted Naumburg's specific importance to art therapy and the uniqueness of art in psychotherapy: "Although Freud had recognized that the unconscious speaks in images, it took art therapy to draw the consequence by making images the final message carrier of the analysis." (p. 4)

Finally, Arnheim concluded:

She was something of an American princess, but the curiously decorative portrait photographs that have been commonly published of her over stress this aspect of her nature. At public occasions to be sure her presence tended to be a formal appearance, but in the practice of her work she was a hard-fisted fighter, pursuing her objectives and defending her principles. To the pleasure of her colleagues and friends she lived to see the fruits of her pioneering. (p. 5)

EDITH KRAMER'S CONTRIBUTION: ART AS THERAPY

Florence Cane's brief comment on the role of the art in psychiatric treatment gives only a hint at a specific method of working. Had she written more we would be able to judge whether her approach was truly at the opposite end of the spectrum from her sister's. But not long after Cane's death Edith Kramer began writing in detail about her own experiences, apparently filling Cane's sisterly role in her focus on the *art* in art therapy.

Austrian-born Kramer

was educated in Vienna and Prague and...studied in Paris. In addition to her formal education in the fine arts, ... Kramer grew up in an atmosphere in which Freudian psychiatry was a dominant intellectual force.... She also studied child psychology at the Psychoanalytic Institute of Prague. ("Introducing...", 1961, p. 5-6)

In the 1930s, Kramer gave art classes in Prague for the children of refugees from Nazi Germany. There she learned of the value of art expression for traumatized children:

> I first observed the different responses to stress as they manifested themselves in children's art, responses that would later become so very familiar to me. I saw regression; repetition that told of unresolved conflict; I first observed identification with the aggressor in children who identified with Hitler, who had proved his power by the very damage he had done to them; I saw withdrawal into frozen rigidity, and, finally, the capacity for creative expression surviving under difficulties. (Kramer, 1971b, p. xiv)

In 1938, just before the Nazis arrived she fled from Czechoslovakia to New York. She worked at settlement houses, schools, and residential programs, including the Wiltwyck School for Boys and the Leake and Watts Children's Home.

> I think of myself as a painter and as an art therapist, not a clinician, an art therapist—which means also understanding something about clinical work but being an art therapist who really uses art as the therapy. It seems to me the

only reason why one would become an art therapist would be that one has something special to offer which only the arts can give. Otherwise you might as well become a psychotherapist.

...

When I came to this country, my first job was at the Little Red Schoolhouse, a progressive elementary school in New York's Greenwich Village. They hired me as a kind of resident shop teacher. They had no money for a shop teacher but they wanted somebody and they figured that a sculptor would be better than a regular carpenter to work with young children. So they thought they might find among those many refugees who came in 1938 a sculptor who could do this work and would live in the building and get his food for free and a little pocket money. And then somehow this became me; I became the tenant of this little room that they had free and started doing some carpentry and sculpture and helped with the clay work and the painting. I mostly did the shop work, which was carpentry, wood carving—we made some marionettes and some masks, besides making bookshelves and footstools and toys. I had done some sculpture so I knew how to handle tools and what I didn't know, I learned on the job—I learned English, too, on the job. I had studied some English before I came, in preparation, so I learned it quickly.

I had this job at Little Red for three years: 1938, '39, '40. Then the war came and I got a job as a machinist in a tool and die factory. I liked it; I did a lot of drawings there. I had an arrangement with the boss that I could punch out after my shift and stay on and draw. That's what kept me

at the job and also I was interested in it. They did origi-
nals; it wasn't a production line job. You got your orders,
your blueprints, and you had to make pieces of metal to
certain specifications. (Kramer in McMahan, 1989, pp.
107–108)

Kramer developed a theory that established for the
growing field a focus opposite that of Naumburg's
(Kramer, 1958). She forcefully postulated the importance of the creative process itself as a healing agent.
These two perspectives established warring camps as the
profession evolved, with followers who often vocifer-
ously argued the merits of their positions. Later training
programs tended to attach themselves to one of the two
theories. The debates continue to this day and contribute
to the liveliness of the field.

Kramer's theoretical model focuses on art *as* therapy,
rather than *in* therapy as Naumburg suggests. Kramer's
stress on the importance of the *art* in art therapy was
something that many art therapists already believed in
and practiced. These art therapists did not refer to themselves as psychotherapists and tended to come, as did
Kramer, from art education.

Kramer's first book, *Art Therapy in a Children's
Community* (1958), described her work from 1951 to
1957 at the Wiltwyck School, a residential treatment

center in New York City for emotionally disturbed boys aged 8 to 12.

At that time you could be poor in America and survive. If I was modest in my demands, I could live on a part-time job and I could continue to paint. I was 33 years old and I figured I had to find something more like a livelihood. People suggested to me that since I was good with kids, particularly the difficult ones, and since I did know a good deal about psychoanalysis and was a good teacher, I should put these together somehow. Dr. Viola Bernard, an analyst, got me a job at the Wiltwyck School for Boys, which was a therapeutic residential community. She was on the professional advisory board and somehow persuaded them to hire me, figuring that I would be able to work with such disturbed children in art.

Q: They hired you as a teacher?

EK: No, actually, I talked to the executive director who said, "Well, what are we going to call what you do?" I said, "Art teaching." "Well," he said, "we are a therapeutic community; everything we do here has to be therapy. We'll call it art therapy."

Q: Was that the first time the term was used?

EK: No, it had been used before by Margaret Naumburg, Adrian Hill, and maybe others. It was not a new word, but I had not really envisioned the work as therapy in that sense. I thought I would work with very difficult kids—difficult, delinquent, wayward children. So I got there and I stayed for 7 years and I did, I think, a very good job and found out how to survive with those kids and how to be useful to them emotionally. (Kramer in McMahan, 1989, p. 108)

In a later book, *Art as Therapy with Children* (1971b), Kramer presented her art therapy programs in residential treatment, in a children's ward of a psychiatric hospital, and in a day school for emotionally disturbed blind children; she further defined her theories.

Although Kramer uses psychoanalytic theory to understand human growth and development and to inform her model of art therapy, she separates the role of the art therapist from that of the psychotherapist in no uncertain terms. Viewing her work as a rather special form of art class, she calls her clients "students" and states that the art therapist must be skilled as artist, teacher, and therapist:

> The art therapist...communicates with his students via the students' paintings and this communication has therapeutic value.... But he is no psychotherapist, and it is not his function to interpret deep unconscious content to his students....
>
> The basic aim of the art therapist is to make available to disturbed persons the pleasures and satisfaction which creative work can give. (Kramer, 1958, p. 5)

Kramer designates art therapy as "an essential component of the therapeutic milieu and a form of therapy which complements or supports psychotherapy *but does not replace it*" (Kramer, 1971b, p. xiii, emphasis added).

> Art therapy is seen as distinct from psychotherapy. Its healing potentialities depend on the psychological processes that are activated in creative work....
>
> [The art therapist] implements the team's therapeutic goals, but he does not ordinarily use his clinical insight for uncovering or interpreting to the patient deep unconscious material, nor does he encourage the development of a transference relationship. (p. 25)

Kramer's theory is based on the psychological processes enhanced by the creative process. Kramer conceives of art therapy as primarily a means of supporting the ego, fostering the development of a sense of identity, and promoting maturation in general. Although she recognizes the role of the unconscious, Kramer cautions that the art therapist "will not, as a rule, directly interpret unconscious meaning, but...will use his knowledge to help the child produce art work that contains and expresses emotionally loaded material" (p. 34).

Not advocating the uncovering of conflicts or the attacking of defenses, Kramer's primary focus is on the use of art to enhance the process of sublimation, which is defined by Freud as a defense mechanism of the ego in which a primitive asocial influence is transformed into a socially productive act.

> It is a process wherein drive energy is deflected from its original goal and displaced onto achievement, which is highly valued by the ego, and is, in most instances, socially productive.... An essential feature of sublimation is the great amount of genuine pleasure the substitute activity affords. (pp. 68–69)

Kramer goes on to make the distinction between substitution and sublimation:

> Substitution which channels actions and emotions without changing their nature remains a safety valve throughout life. When we strike a table with our fist, we express anger, substituting table for person....but this alone is not yet sublimation.
>
> In sublimation we expect a change of the *object* upon which the interest is centered, of the *goal*, and the *kind of energy* through which the goal is achieved. (pp. 70–71, emphasis in the original)

In addition:

> The art therapist's main field of action remains the process of sublimation wherein the material undergoes that final transformation by which it is formed into tangible visual images, and the peculiar fusion between reality and fantasy, between the unconscious and the conscious, which we call art is reached. At this point the art

therapist assists the process by substituting his skill and insight where the student's own resources fail. Since the artistic quality of the production is an indication of the depth and strength of sublimation, the art therapist will encourage a high artistic level of performance within the limitations of the student's talents. (Kramer, 1958, p. 23)

Naumburg de-emphasized the aesthetic nature of the art product and postulated it as a tool for symbolic communication in psychotherapy. Taking a contrasting view, Kramer asserts the importance of the aesthetic quality of the artwork. She believes that the more fully realized and aesthetically pleasing the art, the more complete the sublimation, which to Kramer is the primary goal of art therapy. As the measure of good art, Kramer cites "evocative power, inner consistency, and economy of artistic means" and contends that "the harmony of art is attained through the integration and balance of tensions.... In psychoanalytic terms this harmony is identified with the process of sublimation" (Kramer, 1971b, p. 67).

It is interesting to listen to Edith Kramer's recent observations about the arguments between the grand dames of art therapy theory. She indicates that there may be room to blend aspects of her position with Naumburg's:

[Margaret Naumburg] was giving courses at NYU at that time [1958, the publication of Kramer's first book]. She didn't like me too much because she thought I was really just an art teacher, and I in turn felt that she was more of a psychologist and more a psychotherapist than an art therapist, that she really did not stress art that much. But we later got to know each other better and came to understand each other....

Q: Yours and Margaret Naumburg's points of view have come to represent two divergent lines in art therapy. Do you feel that they're at all beginning to converge again?

EK: Well, I've come to feel that more talk can be included in art therapy than I have included; that there is a place for more psychotherapy in art therapy (under certain circumstances). And I have certainly always felt that one needs psychoanalytic understanding in order to do art therapy; that plain being an artist and a nice person does not suffice to be an art therapist; that you must know what you're dealing with; you must understand the implied and hidden messages. You much know something about illness and health and psychic processes and the unconscious in order to deal with the material that you're getting, because you're getting very heavily loaded material if you ask for it, which you do in the way you set up the whole process. Now, I've always preferred not to talk too much but I've seen other people who talk more and who do very well and it's maybe also a question of temperament. So I would say that there is really no need of seeing it as two opposites with no meeting ground between the two. (Kramer in McMahan, 1989, p. 112)

Despite <u>Naumburg's general acceptance as the "Mother" of art therapy</u>, it should be emphasized that there were a handful of men and women who were at this time also exploring the exciting synergy between art and psychology. Two such people were working in Kansas under the auspices of the Menninger Foundation.

THE MENNINGER FOUNDATION
& CLINIC:
MARY HUNTOON & DON JONES

The Menninger Clinic in Topeka, Kansas, founded in the early 1920s, was a pioneering venture in psychiatric hospital treatment because of its psychoanalytically based, therapeutic milieu. Patients were given long-term, inpatient treatment. Along with psychotherapy, they engaged in a special program of "activities" planned as an adjunct to the therapeutic process. From the beginning, art and music were among these activities. Karl Menninger's interest in and encouragement of the arts is well-known.[6] In 1937, in an article entitled "Encouraging Fantasy Expression in Children," Menninger staff members Jeanetta Lyle[7] and Ruth Faison Shaw, presented a study in which drawings and finger paintings provided access to the child's inner life:

Encouraging the child to draw pictures as a means of facilitating expression of his fantasies, particularly hostile and aggressive ones about which he feels guilt, is a technique frequently used by child analysts and psychologists. The child may say in pictures what he cannot or will not say in words and the analyst can then interpret these drawings in the light of his knowledge of the history of the child's situation. (Lyle & Shaw, 1937, p. 78)

In the 1930s and early 1940s, the Menninger Clinic staff acted as consultants to the Veterans Administration system at a facility called Winter General Hospital. Two art therapists worked at Winter General during this period. Ben Holacher, a ceramicist who used clay primarily with the hundreds of patients he treated, was said to be a gifted, intuitive therapist. Mary Huntoon, a printmaker and artist, was hired by Menninger to work in the VA system. She was born in Topeka, Kansas, in 1896 and studied under artist George Stone and others at Washburn University in Topeka. Upon graduating in 1920, she moved to New York City and studied at the Art Students League with Joseph Pennell, Robert Henri, and George Bridgeman. A year later Huntoon left for Paris to create etchings for a New York publishing syndicate. She remained in France for 5 years and had her first one-person show at the Galerie Sacre du Printemps in 1929. In 1930, Huntoon returned to Topeka, and in 1933, she assumed the directorship of the Federal Arts Project until 1938. She headed the activity program in 1936 at the Menninger Sanitarium which included sketching and painting and was an art instructor from 1935 to 1938. Her job description changed from "instructor" to "therapist" in 1949, and to "manual arts therapist" in 1956 (Junge, 1987). It was in 1935, according to Hagaman (1986), that Karl Menninger asked Huntoon to introduce work in visual arts into patients' therapy at the hospital. She called herself an art therapist and evolved a way of working that she termed "dynamically oriented art therapy." What Huntoon meant by this term was that she worked according to her knowledge of the psychodynamics of the case, but she did not use a psychotherapeutic approach. In an activity program for Menninger's (circa 1935–1936) she outlined her treatment using art:

A. Methods of Approach
    1. Diagnosis: Spontaneous approach to art for diagnosis purposes.
    2. As therapy—skills, dexterity (occupational treatment).

B. Art therapy as release of creative process
    1. Personality is to experience the creative process.

2. Patient's hopes, fears and conflicts are expressed.
3. Patient also has a better understanding after he has painted his idea or problem.

C. The mind may become bent but the creative faculty remains unbent. (memo from the Huntoon Archives, no date)

As early as 1934, Huntoon joined an art therapy program under the direction of Ruth Shaw who introduced finger painting as therapy. Huntoon joined the faculty of the Psychiatric Training Program at the Winter Veterans Administration Hospital in Topeka, and stayed on in various capacities until the late 1950s.[8] Once at the VA she established and directed the Department of Art, Physical Medicine, and Rehabilitation (Figure 1).[9] In a letter to a friend, Huntoon said of her new position:

> Another thing has meant remaining in Topeka...it seemed both wise and an opportunity to accept the position offered to me as head of the art shop of the Medicine and Rehabilitation Department at the Winter VA Hospital. This work in the field of art therapy was not new to me because of my work at the Menninger Foundation some 10 years before where I had taught art twice a week for over 3 years. I have built up the art shop so that it is considered one of the leading efforts in the particular field, I handle almost two dozen art mediums [sic]...and correlate my department with the psychiatric and psychology

departments of the hospital. (letter dated August 21, 1947, Huntoon Archives)

While at the VA, Huntoon focused on research (Figure 2) which provided the basis for several papers including: "The Creative Arts as Therapy" (1949), "Art Therapy for Patients in the Acute Section of Winter VA Hospital" (1953), and "Art for Therapy's Sake" (1959). She later returned to the Menninger Foundation as faculty to teach marriage counseling from 1953 to 1960. Mary Huntoon died of cancer in 1970 at age 74.

Huntoon retired 10 years before the American Art Therapy Association was founded, but she had been active in another professional organization. She was a founding member of the American Association of Rehabilitation Therapists (AART) and presented on art therapy at its first conference. She also served as the chair of the AART research committee which funded art therapy studies (Hagaman, 1986, p. 95).

In 1938, Margaret Naumburg was invited to give a presentation on art therapy at the Menninger Clinic. Apparently, she clashed with Karl Menninger and left before her presentation. However, it is known that she met and talked with Mary Huntoon. Robert Ault (1985) told the perhaps apocryphal story of this meeting and suggested that Naumburg might have "borrowed" Huntoon's terminology because it was soon after her meeting with Huntoon that Naumburg began to define what she did as "dynamically oriented art therapy" and published her ideas. Another connection between the two women occurred in 1954, when Naumburg asked Huntoon to send patient work for an exhibit titled "Use of Spontaneous Art in Psychotherapy." However, Huntoon's work was not included because, according to Naumburg, there was "no space" (Huntoon Archives, no date).

While Huntoon did publish some articles and make professional presentations, her work was not well-known nationally. It was only much later that she attended a conference of the American Art Therapy Association. Thus her presence and activity as a pioneering art therapist were largely invisible to her colleagues. She is perhaps representative of others working as artists or art teachers or even art therapists in special settings in the 1930s and 1940s, whose labors have largely gone unsung. Huntoon said:

> Art can help the mending. The psychotic, completely withdrawn from reality; the psychoneurotic, knowing the aberrations within himself and still needing help in adjustment; any individual with a bent mind, if his creative

faculty remains intact, can be helped. He may not be able to talk, but he can still paint....

Research in what art can do for the mentally ill is still in the pioneer stage. I certainly don't know all its possibilities; I doubt if anyone does. But we'll find out someday and meantime, the great help it gives our patients right now more than justifies our faith in it. (Huntoon, 1948, p. 23)

During the Second World War, Don Jones registered as a conscientious objector and was assigned to work at Marlboro State Psychiatric Hospital in New Jersey in 1942. Committed to working with people since high school, he had hoped to find a way to combine his interests in art and theology. At the hospital, Jones noticed that art seemed to hold great meaning for the patients: "I immediately became intrigued by the many graphic productions and projections of patients which literally covered the walls of some rooms and of passageways between different buildings" (Jones in Levick, 1983a, p. 6).

Between 1942 and 1946, Jones collected hundreds of drawings and paintings by patients. Adding drawings of his own, he put them together in a book about state hospital life called *PRN* (Civilian Public Service Unit, 1946). During his 4 years at the psychiatric hospital,

Mary Huntoon   221 Huntoon Street——Studio   Topeka Kansas

September 3, 1947

Ruth Mannoni (Mrs. S.A),
412 N. Grant,
Chanute, Kansas

Dear Mrs. Mannoni:

The Public Relations Department of the Winter VA Hospital has sent
your letter of August 25th, 1947, inquiring about the Art Therapy work
in Kansas, to me as head of the Art Department Therapy here. I shall
send you our program, hoping that it will answer some of your questions.
Under Dr. Karl and Dr. Will Menninger's management we have been able to
do pioneering work in this field, and the Executive Director of the
Rehabilitation program, Miss Edna Vehlow, has given me a free hand in
my department's development. We call the field that of creative and
intuitional therapy.

In the accompanying pages I have tried to give you an over-view of the
work being accomplished. Since April 10th. 1946, when we had nothing
but a few drafting table ans one easel, we have built up a department
which can present the student with twenty media, thus giving range
for almost any personality adjustment. At the present time we are
correlating our program with that of the psychological and psychiatric
departments for more effective therapy. This is a new field and
one which is very inspiring in the results of our individual therapy.
We treat neurological, the purely physical, psychotic, and neurotic
is prescribed by the doctor. A patient is prescribed to Art Therapy
if there is either Art experience in his background or the need of
creative therapy for his illness.

                    Sincerely yours,

                              Mary Huntoon, Supervisor
                              Art Department,
                              Manual Arts Section,
                              Physical. ed. Rehab.
                              Winter VA Hospital
                              Topeka,
                              Kansas

Figure 1

CREATIVE ARTS THERAPY SHOWING CLINICAL CLASSIFICATION
OF ART USED AS TREATMENT

PURPOSE OF RESEARCH   To define the role of Arts in the treatment of many types of mental illness, in which an exploratory period has already been given to the study of certain types, using the studio as a laboratory in which rehabilitation and motivation of these types has already been observed.

OBJECTIVES OF RESEARCH   To re-examine and re-evaluate the material studied, and to tabulate all material gained in the clinical study of the use of Art as treatment for many types of mental illness for both open and closed ward patients. To systematize this material and to correlate the studio productions with the progress in the rehabilitation of the patients treated.

INTRODUCTION   The development of treatment techniques through clinical experience afforded by the use of Art as adjunctive therapy in Physical Medicine Rehabilitation has resulted in the observation of material which has remained unsystematized, and unavailable to the general field of rehabilitation. The need for criteria and techniques which the physician may use is apparent in both the rehabilitation program and in vocational guidance. As projective phenomena studio production have value in a field in which it is almost impossible to give conclusive tests, i.e. tests cannot be conclusively given which show whether or not a patient has, through the use of his sensitive faculty, collected material which may be expressed graphically, and which may through the use of his latent creative faculty, aid in his rehabilitation. the use of the studio as a testing laboratory had yielded material otherwise unattainable.

THE ROLE OF ART USED AS TREATMENT   The creative process itself is therapeutic, engaging the patient in his own recovery as well as affording material which may aid his doctor in formulating the treatment necessary for his rehabilitation.

WORKING ARRANGEMENTS   The estimated cost of the research should cover a full-time salary for an assistant instructor, and a full-time secretary, as well as the half-time salary of the supervisor of the program, the supervisor remaining as half-time employee of the Art shop in order to relate the shop as a laboratory for observation. The cost of materials already used which will become part of the research material should be reimbursed and transferred and the cost of new materials which will become necessary in re-cataloging and re-evaluating the material, must be estimated. Racks will be necessary for the catalogued paintings, and all material should be published in some permanent form for referral. At least nine categories are indicated in the grouping of material into those already found in the use of art as treatment. The estimated cost of such a research for one year is from $12,00 to $15,000. Much of the work has been indicated by the laboratory work already done by the present supervisor of Creative Arts Therapy, and it is suggested that half of her time be devoted to the research project, directing the cataloguing. One full-time instructor for the research laboratory work, and one full-time secretary for the cataloguing and assembling of all material.

It is proposed to take selected patient for the project, showing the manner in which their works falls into certain art categories, with correlating of categories to media used, and the exposing of patients to form and color in determining method of carrying out the prescribed aim. It is also proposed to show the supportive therapy role as related to the laboratory changes shown in the work of the patient.

The nine categories already selected:

1. Fantasy and wish-fulfillment
2. Dexterity-facade
3. Drainage-painting out-catharsis
4. Dreams
5. Conflict painting
6. Ego integration and externalization
7. Color dynamics
8. The use of Art on the Child Level for the Acutely Ill who are without special art ability.
9. Ego Persistence shown by use of Art in Pre-and Post-lobotomy

Figure 2 (cont.)

47

Jones painted as a catharsis for himself. A later manuscript, *Tunnel*, (Jones, 1947) contained Jones's paintings about the patients he had worked with.

Teaching art classes in Kansas in 1950, Jones's students were psychiatrists and social workers from the Menninger Clinic. Through them he was introduced to Karl Menninger. Enthusiastic about the manuscript, Menninger wanted the artwork for the Menninger Museum. According to Jones,

> Menninger said "I must have these paintings for the Menninger Museum." I wrote Dr. Karl a letter saying that you must have Don Jones also if you're going to have his paintings.... You need me to do art therapy, whatever that is. (Jones, 1975)

Jones came to work at the Menninger Clinic in 1951 and began to develop what was to become an extensive expressive arts program which employed and trained many art therapists. Originally an adjunctive activities therapy, art therapy was offered in later years as a form of psychotherapy and was one of the psychotherapy options available to patients. Jones stayed on at the clinic until 1966 when he went to Harding Hospital in Worthington, Ohio, as Director of the Adjunctive Therapy Department. Although Jones had had extensive art training in high school, the war had interrupted his college plans. Jones reflected: "The state hospital was my university of psychiatry and Menninger's later gave me the words to explain the experiences that I had.... At Menninger's I translated my experiential knowledge of mental patients to some theoretical base" (Jones, 1975).

Jones has presented widely and published his work on art therapy with hospitalized patients (Jones, 1962). In the early years, he made a particular effort to connect with art educators and spoke at many of their conferences. He was one of the first art therapists to treat persons with multiple personality disorder, contributing to our knowledge of that once rare and fascinating syndrome.

PARALLEL DEVELOPMENTS
Hidden Art Therapists

Many of the first art therapists did not write about their work or give national presentations as did Naumburg. Consequently, there is little documentation available to reconstruct the history of the field in the 1940s and 1950s. Some individuals began as art teachers in special settings and gradually developed methods which suited the groups with which they worked. Few called themselves "art therapists." A number began in volunteer positions which only later developed into paying positions. Some were convinced they were the only ones doing what they did and were surprised to find any compatriots let alone specific books or articles on the subject.

Relatively unknown art therapists included people such as Prentiss Taylor and Georgette Powell in Washington, DC; Dorothy Royer, Tobe Reisel, and Christine Sharpes in California; Myer Site in Baltimore, Maryland; Edith Zierer, her husband Ernest, and Clara Jo Stember in New York; and Edythe Polsby Salzberger in Texas. Unfortunately, there are others whose names are lost to history.

Art Therapy in England

We should note that the development of art therapy in England parallels that of art therapy in the United States. For example, as in the United States, the tradition of artists rather than medical professionals or paraprofessionals becoming art therapists pervaded. According to Waller (1992), the term "art therapy" has been used in Great Britain since the late 1930s, and it is included within the National Health Service. Waller identifies the roots of British art therapy in psychoanalysis, developmental psychology, occupational therapy, and art education (specifically Franz Cizek's ideas about child art). During World War II both group psychotherapy and art therapy evolved.

Adrian Hill takes credit for coining the term "art therapy" in 1942 (Hill, 1951, p. 13). Hill, a professional artist who was recovering in a tuberculosis sanatorium, turned to his art for his own therapy and subsequently received permission to introduce painting to other patients (Hill, 1948; 1951). He discovered that the patients both enjoyed the work and used it to express their feelings, fears, and the traumatic occurrences of the war. Also in 1942, Rita Simon, a commercial artist, conducted art sessions for outpatient groups under the auspices of Joshua Bierer who had begun "social psychiatry clubs." Waller writes that: "Simon quickly became aware of the potential for using art as a means of expression and communication and entered her own psychoanalysis in order to understand more about the therapeutic process" (Waller, 1992, p. 8).

The artist Edward Adamson was hired in 1946 at Netherne Psychiatric Hospital to aid medical staff in research into the effects of leucotomy on visual perception. Later he developed paintings for diagnosing specific disorders[10] and established a gallery of patients' artwork at Netherne. *Art as Healing* (1984) describes Adamson's work and mentions that he had done some early work with Adrian Hill. Frank Breakwell, one of Hill's pupils, helped to form the British Art Therapy Association in 1964. During this time, Jungian psychoanalyst Irene Champernowne and her husband established the Withymead Centre for Psychotherapy Through the Arts, a private clinic in Devon, England.[11] As Waller states,

> In the 1960s and early 1970s, it appears that art therapy practice was not unlike a sensitive form of art teaching—similar to that of the best art colleges where the therapist took care to encourage the patients to develop their own form of visual expression and entered into a supportive, nonconfrontative relationship. Art therapy departments tended to be somewhat isolated from the rest of the hospital, and therapists worked on their own.... Although some founder art therapists had experience of psychotherapy themselves or had some training in psychology, it was not until the late 1970s and early 1980s that some of them developed a stronger orientation toward psychodynamic practice. (Waller, 1992, p. 89)

The Early Relationship Between Art Therapy & the Psychiatric Community

An important outcome of Don Jones's tenure at Menninger's was that art therapy began to be more visible because of its connection to a prestigious institution and because of the psychiatrists, mental health staff, and visitors who saw it in action there. As a visual medium, art therapy has had the advantage of having its attributes more visible and obvious than many of the other therapies During the 1940s, 1950s, and 1960s, Margaret Naumburg often spent time introducing dynamically oriented art therapy to professional groups such as psychiatrists, psychologists, art educators, and to the staffs of medical schools and psychiatric hospitals as well as the general public. She also produced art therapy exhibits for professional conferences, museums, and other institutions both in the United States and in Europe.

In 1954, Réné Spitz, an outstanding Freudian analyst, served as the chief discussant at a symposium on art therapy at the American Orthopsychiatric Association meeting in New York City. He began by describing his use of art with several of his patients who had difficulty talking. Spitz's patients made paintings in the presence of an art teacher he had employed for the purpose. She offered art supplies but was instructed specifically to make no comments. The patients brought their art to Spitz at their next analytic session. Spitz saw fundamental differences between classical psychoanalysis and art therapy:

While in analytical therapy the analyst remains anonymous, non-interfering, does not manipulate the patient and stays extremely passive, the situation in art therapy by its very nature is completely different. Art therapy, of necessity takes place in a social situation. The therapist has to manipulate the patient to a certain extent; the therapist has to interfere to a certain extent and can by no means remain as passive and certainly not as anonymous as the analyst. (Réné Spitz, quoted in Naumburg, 1966, p. 17)

Naumburg quarreled with Spitz's viewpoint calling it "a misunderstanding," and she particularly rankled at the word "manipulation." She pointed out that patient artworks are not always produced in the presence of the art therapist but can be made at home or in the psychiatric hospital and brought to the therapist. She emphasized that art therapy not only included spontaneous expression through pictures but also verbal communication between patient and art therapist, focusing on problems and conflicts (Naumburg, 1966, pp. 17–18).

Thus, it is important to recognize that the early growth of the art therapy profession came in large measure because of this cross-fertilization between art therapy and the psychiatric community. Art therapists early on took the opportunity to tell others about their work. In addition to describing what happened in the sessions, they showed the patients' artwork; the audience could see in a compelling and convincing way, the concrete visual record of the power and potential of art in therapy. In almost every case, early art therapists were helped by psychiatrists and psychoanalysts who were directors of hospitals or institutes (such as Karl Menninger and Nolan D. C. Lewis) or in private practice and who, because of their deep personal interest in art and their awareness of the psychological processes that art could evoke, were willing to experiment. They offered fledgling art therapists employment, opportunities to practice and to publish, and gave art therapy a kind of validity within the psychiatric community it might not have otherwise achieved for years to come.

In the 1950s, there was a proliferation of writings by art therapists which increased notice of the new discipline across the country. Margaret Naumburg published *Schizophrenic Art: Its Meaning in Psychotherapy* (1950) and *Psychoneurotic Art: Its Function in Psychotherapy* (1953). In 1958, Naumburg contributed a chapter ("Art Therapy: Its Scope and Function") and a case study ("Art Therapy with a Seventeen-Year-Old Schizophrenic Girl") to Emanuel F. Hammer's *The Clinical Application of Projective Drawings*. In Hammer's book, Lauretta Bender, John Buck, and Karen Machover, among others, provided the collaboration of clinicians and researchers in a comprehensive exploration of projective drawings used in diagnosis and therapy. The book also offered increased visibility to Margaret Naumburg and to art therapy.

In Houston, Texas, Irving Kraft, then Chief of Child Psychiatry at Houston State Psychiatric Hospital, read Naumburg's work and suggested to his friend Felice Cohen that they use this modality in the treatment of their patients (Cohen, 1975a). Cohen, a fourth generation Texan, had been interested in psychology in college and attended two years of medical school. She later got a degree in bacteriology and, at the time she began work with Kraft, called herself a "Sunday painter." Her contributions as an art therapist have been informed by a bent for research, and her work has included topics such as art therapy with the transsexual patient (Cohen, 1976), the introduction of art therapy into the public schools (Cohen, 1975b), and most recently, a study of graphic indicators in the artwork of child-abuse victims (Cohen & Phelps, 1985).

Tarmo Pasto had been a Professor of Art and Psychology at Sacramento State College (originally called California State College at Sacramento) since 1950. With an $80,000 grant from the National Institute of Mental

Health, he conducted a research project from 1963 to 1965, categorizing graphic imagery of institutionalized mental patients and also those in the California Youth Authority programs and State Department of Corrections (Holden, 1965). The grant also funded a publication *Ars Gratia Hominis*[12] which Pasto and Peter Runkel edited. Pasto wrote that artists had abrogated their role of providing "the one great means of experiencing emotion.... However, in the hands of two of society's most inarticulate groups, the artistic object remained a direct manifestation of inner meaning. These two groups, whose art productions have been 'discovered' only recently, are children and the insane" (Pasto, 1962, p. 73).

It was Pasto's conviction that:

A true work of art functions on several psychological levels: (1) as a projection of the body-image, it reflects one's view of the self in a world of objects and therefore provides a means of self-identification and confrontation; (2) it ascribes a meaning to and develops an understanding of the objective world; (3) it provides an outlet for expression of unconscious images; (4) it provides a language that deals more lucidly with emotional meanings than the more conscious conceptual written or spoken word; and (5) it provides for ego-development through the conscious effort required in manipulation of both images and materials. (pp. 73–74)

As to the function of the art therapist, Pasto described how:

> The art therapist does not need to criticize pictures from an academic point of view, or bring in principles of art, but must rather draw out from the patient answers to such questions as: Is this the color you felt best expressed the idea? Is there more than one idea involved? How can you clarify this as to placement in space? What does a tree mean to you? Is the mountain heavy or light? Are there shadows? Is the sun shining? The idea is to keep the patient thinking about and clarifying on a perceptual-motor level the emotional experience out of which the image developed. (p. 74)

But as for specific interpretations of art or the actual mechanism by which the art therapy process helped patients, Pasto had to admit he had few answers:

> One can see that the art therapist is dealing with many complex things. Often both he and the patient will forever remain in the dark as to what the art expression means, or why art expression assisted the patient to recovery. (p. 76)

Pasto was instrumental in the careers of two art therapists in Northern California, Donald Uhlin and Cay Drachnik. Don Uhlin had studied with Viktor Lowenfeld and worked with Pasto in his studies of prisoners and their artwork. Uhlin became a professor of art and later started an art therapy program at California State College at Sacramento. Cay Drachnik was the first graduate. She had moved to California in 1972 from Northern Virginia, a suburb of Washington, DC, where she had taken one course from Elinor Ulman and a weekend course from Christine Wang, another Washington art therapist. In 1973, she convinced Uhlin to start the program at the state university. She writes, "I think later it helped in political issues when we could say that art therapists were not only trained in private colleges.... Legislators respond to that" (Drachnik, 1992, p. 4).

Elinor Ulman & the Creation of the First Art Therapy Journal

In the early 1950s, Elinor Ulman, living in Washington, DC, organized a lecture series for Margaret Naumburg. Ulman had graduated from Wellesley College as as Phi Beta Kappa with a Bachelor of Arts in English literature. After college she studied painting with Maurice Sterne, George Grosz, and Othon Coubine and Chinese brush painting in Peiping (now Bei-jing), China. Her paintings were exhibited at the Corcoran

Biennial, Pennsylvania Academy, New York's World's Fair of 1939, and the Phillips Memorial Gallery among others. She developed "a passionate interest in landscape," obtained a Bachelor of Science in landscape architecture from Iowa State College and worked as a landscape architect and draftsperson (Ulman, 1971; "Introducing...", 1961, p. 2). Ulman says: "I drifted into art therapy by a rather round about road but at the time I drifted in there weren't any direct roads" (Ulman, 1975a).

> Actually, I was already working in art therapy when I helped arrange the series of lectures in Washington by Margaret Naumburg. Mostly, I read a lot and [was helped by] the somewhat unconventional teaching at the American University in art education with an artist Robin Bond.... I put it all together and took the plunge. I volunteered at several different places and made it up as I went along. Besides Margaret Naumburg, some of the innovative art educators like Florence Cane and Henry Schaefer-Simmern were very influential on my teaching of art and I really thought [what I was doing] was teaching art. (Ulman, 1975a)

In 1951, planning to teach art, Ulman joined her friend Jeannie McConnell Cannon who was working with children at a special school and in a child guidance clinic in England for what she called "an apprenticeship."

After returning to Washington, Ulman worked as a volunteer with neurologically handicapped children and in an alcohol clinic and then took a position in a psychiatric unit of the District of Columbia General Hospital, where she practiced for 10 years. She also took courses at the Washington School of Psychiatry. In 1957, she became a faculty member there. It was at DC General that Ulman met Bernard I. Levy, the Chief Psychologist, who taught her the principles of research and psychiatric diagnosis. During this time she developed what is now called the Ulman Personality Assessment Procedure (Ulman, 1975b). The two became life-long friends. Levy, an ebullient painter of peaceful watercolors, became Chair of the Department of Psychology at the George Washington University. With Ulman, he founded the art therapy program there in 1971. Although Levy[13] was the Director, the program was always clearly a joint work, as, in many ways, would be the creation of a professional journal.

Ulman made important contributions to the field of art therapy as a writer and editor. In her writing she attempted both to describe and understand the process of art therapy and to explore and extend definitions of the field. However, unquestionably her major contribution was the creation of *The Bulletin of Art Therapy* in 1961, the first and, until 1973, only journal in the field.

In 1970, shortly after the organization of the American Art Therapy Association (AATA), Ulman renamed her publication *The American Journal of Art Therapy* (AJAT) which seemed to indicate an official connection to the American Art Therapy Association, causing some confusion. AATA's *Newsletter,* edited at the time by Don Jones, immediately issued the following disclaimer:

> The recent change of name of *The Bulletin* to *The American Journal of Art Therapy* does not imply that this journal in any way is related to AATA. It is privately subsidized and edited. The *Newsletter* is the only publication which speaks for AATA and its membership. (Jones, 1970)

Conceived originally as a newsletter by Ulman and Bernard Levy, it quickly became a journal. According to Ulman, "Edith Kramer agreed to do a lead article for the first issue. We found one book to review and that's how we started" (Ulman, 1975a). In her first editorial Ulman set forth her goals:

> Above all, we look forward to rigorous intellectual debate as the only road to meaningful consensus. The most cre-

ative thinkers often wage battles over ideas that seem to them irreconcilable. When the dust has settled, eclectic minds wonder at the passionate controversy over separate facets of a single truth. But clarity and depth of understanding will not result from a superficial glossing over of differences.... We trust that from readers deeply concerned with art, education, and psychotherapy we shall get expressions characterized by the liveliness, force, and disciplined freedom that are the common goal we seek for our patients, our students, and ourselves (Ulman, 1961a, p. 5).

Controversy would become one of Ulman's signatures. In 1974, Ulman's journal became officially affiliated with the American Art Therapy Association. However, AATA members spent considerable time in annual meetings discussing the pros and cons of this affiliation. Most of the controversy centered on the choice of book reviewers, AATA representation on the editorial board, and subsidies of the journal through membership dues.[14] Ulman defended her high editorial standards while some members thought such standards were a means for controlling or excluding certain authors. Ten years later upon the lapse of the contract, after considerable antagonism and acrimony, and unable to reach a satisfactory agreement for AATA to take over ownership, *The American Journal of Art Therapy* and AATA separated. After 23 years as editor and publisher of AJAT, Ulman agreed that Vermont College of Norwich University in Montpelier, Vermont, would own and publish the journal. Barbara Sobol served briefly as the editor in 1985–1986, and Gladys Agell became editor in 1986; but Ulman remained its executive editor until her death in 1991.[15] Linda Gantt commented:

> Many members of AATA did not realize that Elinor funded *AJAT* from the beginning and that subscriptions never paid for the operation. She personally absorbed substantial losses many (if not most) years. She was reluctant to talk about money and especially reluctant to raise subscription rates to break even. Given her resistance to publicize her own financial contributions it is little wonder that most members had no idea that her "control" of *AJAT* was justified to her since she footed the bill. (Gantt, 1991, personal communication)

Speaking of her motivation in starting the journal, Ulman said she thought that one day, art therapists

> would begin to get organized. I decided that I would like to be an organizer rather than an organizee. What was partly in the back of my mind in founding the journal was that writing and editing were close to my heart. I also thought correctly that it would put me in a position, when an organization began to happen—it would put me in the middle of things. (Ulman, 1975a)

Elinor Ulman's founding of *The Bulletin of Art Therapy* was of immense importance and created a tremendous impetus for the evolving profession. People who had been working alone in different areas of the country, sometimes calling what they did art therapy, sometimes not, found that there were others like them engaged in the exciting endeavor of using art for therapeutic purposes. In later years, citing their loneliness as solitary art therapists, many would remember the journal as a lifeline. Ulman presented current thinking on a variety of aspects in the field and articles by clinicians on their work that was swiftly evolving to include not only therapy with the individual patient, but also with groups and, by the late 1960s, even with families. She printed news on events by and for art therapists, book reviews (often by Bernard Levy), film reviews, and letters to the editor. Her editorials were occasionally argumentative and vehement but spoke of a passion for the field that was beginning to be shared by many. Elinor Ulman herself remained a figure of controversy in the evolution of organized art therapy. She was right in her conviction that the creation of the journal would put her in the middle of things. A woman of intelligence and strong opinions, she was often seen as obstructionist and divisive:

I was opposed to the Association in the beginning, because I didn't think it was time to establish an organization. But of course, if people like me had been in charge, the Association probably never would have happened. So I have to admit, maybe it was a good thing, that some go-getters got in there and plunged ahead. (Ulman in Jordan, 1988, p. 109)

She has always fought tenaciously and vehemently for her views. When asked if there were any "negative consequences" from her involvement with the Association, Ulman replied:

Fights. I think I have a reputation of being a fighter. In fact, I was accused of liking to fight, and I don't think I like to fight. But when doing what I want to do involves a fight, I'd rather go down fighting than give up. If I lose a battle, I lose a battle. But if I don't fight, then I always think I might have won. ... I learned to be more indirect, that if you come out and say what you mean—and especially if you make wisecracks with some punch to them—that you cause more anger than enlightenment. So I've learned to be not quite so openly attacking. But in one of the early issues there was an account of the first annual conference of the Association,[16] and it was very sarcastic. I enjoy being sarcastic when I'm really angry—so there are some things about fighting that I like.

Q. How was your sarcasm received?

Ulman: With rage. We got some very angry letters. (Ulman in Jordan, 1988, p. 109)

However, for more than 30 years, Ulman's journal contributed in an extraordinarily important way as a vehicle of communication for art therapists of all philosophical backgrounds. Indeed, without Ulman's farsightedness in creating a national publication to give voice to art therapy, it is quite likely that the professional organization and the profession would have been much longer in its creation. Ulman published two anthologies of articles from the journal (Ulman & Dachinger, 1975; Ulman & Levy, 1980). With Edith Kramer and Hanna Yaxa Kwiatkowska, she wrote the monograph *Art Therapy in the United States* (1978), but as Edith Kramer said after Ulman's death:

> Alas, Elinor spoke too seldom. Suffering from severe writer's block, she never wrote the books she ought to have written...a loss to the profession. The block, however, made her a superb editor. It was the gain of the many who contributed to the *Bulletin* and later to *AJAT* as well as the gain of the countless students whose papers she mercilessly corrected. (Kramer, 1992a, p. 67)

The journal's 1961 birth was the landmark event which both signaled the end of art therapy's "formative years" and gave it the essential vehicle it needed to move forward. After that would come a period of expansion and consolidation for art therapy, based at least in part, on the foundation stones laid by Ulman.

HANNA YAXA KWIATKOWSKA: THE CREATION OF FAMILY ART THERAPY

Another who attended Naumburg's lectures in Washington along with Elinor Ulman was Hanna Yaxa Kwiatkowska. Kwiatkowska, an artist and sculptor trained in her native Poland, fled during the second World War to Brazil where she continued her successful artistic career. She spoke seven languages fluently and was educated in Switzerland, Austria, and Warsaw. She came to the United States and eventually met Margaret Naumburg. Aware of her need for a solid training in psychology, psychiatry, and psychoanalysis, Kwiatkowska attended the William Alanson White Institute in New York. There she studied under such teachers as Clara Thompson and Erich Fromm.

Kwiatkowska began her first experiments in art therapy from 1955 to 1958 at St. Elizabeths Hospital in Washington where, as she wrote "with no official title, I was given the freedom to design my own programs" (Kwiatkowska, 1978, p. xiii). At St. Elizabeths, Kwiatkowska used art with groups of patients and designed the research project "A Blind Study of the Influence of Chlorpromazine (Thorazine) on Graphic Expression of Schizophrenic Patients." Through a meeting with the well-known psychoanalyst Frieda Fromm-Reichmann, she joined the staff at the National Institute of Mental Health (NIMH) in 1958 under Drs. Lyman C. Wynne and Juliana Day Franz, where she remained for 14 years.

Kwiatkowska joined NIMH at an extraordinarily fruitful period of research into the etiology of schizophrenia which helped provide important clinical information on families and launched much of the family therapy movement as we know it today. Murray Bowen, who had worked first at the Menninger Foundation and then at NIMH in the early 1950s, arranged for family members to be hospitalized along with the schizophrenic patient in order to study the family unit. Lyman Wynne, who succeeded Bowen as Director of the Family Studies Section at NIMH, centered his research on the confused and confusing patterns of communication in families with schizophrenic members. At first, Kwiatkowska treated individual patients. Then employing art as a research tool to assess families, she realized that the art could also be used as treatment to help a family's communication and enable them to recognize and work on dynamics. She evolved a six-step procedure for the evaluation of a family that dramatically exemplified the usefulness of art in assessment. The set of drawings which Kwiatkowska elicited from family members consisted of:

1. A free picture[17]
2. A picture of your family
3. An abstract family portrait
4. A picture started with the help of a scribble[18]
5. A joint family scribble
6. A free picture. (Kwiatkowska, 1978, p. 86)

This particular sequence of pictures was important because Kwiatkowska believed that the move from freedom to more structure exerted increasing stress on the family members. Thus a comparison of the last free picture with the first and a reading of their messages provided Kwiatkowska an indication of how the family handled the stress of the session. After each drawing, family members were encouraged to observe and comment on each other's work. Kwiatkowska also integrated verbal and art therapy by the simple but innovative suggestion that the family's primary therapist work with her as a co-therapist.

Kwiatkowska's first paper was on her work with an individual and was published in 1959 as "A

Schizophrenic Patient's Response in Art Therapy to Changes in the Life of the Psychotherapist" (Kwiatkowska & Perlin, 1959). Kwiatkowska's important work with families was published in articles throughout the 1960s (Day & Kwiatkowska, 1962; Kwiatkowska, Day, & Wynne, 1962; Kwiatkowska, 1962, 1967) but did not appear as a book until 1978 with the publication of *Family Therapy and Evaluation Through Art*. "As an artist, she worked and exhibited in Switzerland, Austria, Manchuria and Brazil, as well as the United States" (Gantt, 1991, personal communication). She was granted 3 Fulbright travel awards to lecture in Brazil. This was the first time that the United States government sponsored information about art therapy as part of its scientific exchange. While in Brazil, her knowledge of Portuguese enabled her to do a family art therapy demonstration with a Brazilian couple, their daughter and schizophrenic son. ("News...", 1965, pp. 74-76)

Kwiatkowska was an assistant professor of art therapy at the George Washington University and a visiting professor at the Catholic University of Rio de Janeiro, Brazil. She died in 1980.[19] Her student and colleague, art therapist Harriet Wadeson wrote movingly of her experience with Kwiatkowska in these excerpts from the poem "The Last Lesson":

...

In the long-ago maze of being teacher and student
we used to speak of luscious delicacies,
profiteroles, pâté, Amaretto soufflé.
We passed each other symbols
of the exotic nourishment we craved....

...

I didn't repeat what you had taught me
because I had not yet fully learned it.

I still see your fragile face fluttering in the wind,
the deep sigh in your dark eyes,
and the canes and crutches[20] of all those years.
And only now,
three years since that last goodbye,
plowing a field where your students and mine
have become planters,
do I reap the full harvest of your teachings.
The wind roars the name of the last lesson:
Courage.

(Wadeson, 1982, p. 124)

BEGINNING STEPS IN
ART THERAPY EDUCATION

Formal education in art therapy began in the 1950s. First came Naumburg's many presentations, which fascinated mental health professionals and those interested in the emerging field. Some art therapists such as Naumburg, Ulman, and Kwiatkowska took classes at psychoanalytic institutes and schools of psychiatry which helped to give other professionals a look at art therapists and art therapy through class discussions. Naumburg's training seminars in "The Techniques and Methods of Art Therapy" were given in the early 1950s in New York, Philadelphia, Washington, and Cambridge, Massachusetts, and often led to requests for more information on the new therapeutic discipline. Ulman remembers, "After her lectures, people would ask Margaret Naumburg where they could hear more. Much to our surprise we heard her say 'Hanna Kwiatkowska and Elinor Ulman could give more training so they'll do it'" (Ulman, 1975a).

After that, Ulman developed and taught art therapy courses to psychiatrists, social workers, and nurses at the Washington School of Psychiatry from 1957 until 1973. Margaret Naumburg states that in 1958, she presented "the first training program which dealt with the principles and methods of dynamically oriented art therapy" for graduate students in a university setting (Naumburg, 1966, p. 31). The course, "Art Education and Personality," was given in the Department of Art Education at New York University. It is of interest that, despite Naumburg's own clinical emphasis on art in psychotherapy, this pioneer in education presented her first academic course not in a department of psychology or the like, but in an art education department and with an art education title. Perhaps this is not so odd if we remember her passion for progressive education.

A year earlier, in 1957, the University of Louisville had initiated a Master's degree program in art therapy. Originating in the Psychology Department and the Art Department, the program had no art therapist to coordinate it. Nevertheless, it graduated two students in 1959. After that, the program remained more or less inactive until 1969 when Sandra Kagin,[21] a 25-year-old art therapist who had moved to Louisville from Kansas, called to talk with Roger White about the program. He told her that there was no program at that time and asked if she would like to get it started again. Kagin was hired by the University of Louisville the same day in June, 1969, that art therapists, invited by White to the

Louisville campus, initiated the fledgling American Art Therapy Association.

Beginning in 1960, Roy Stern and Harold Winn gave a course called "Psychiatric Art Therapy" at Temple University School of Medicine, Department of Psychiatry. Starting with a course taught here and there, the next 25 years would see the proliferation of introductory courses across the country and then the development of graduate-school, institute, and clinical programs. In addition, standards in education and training for art therapists would be developed to parallel and eventually equal those in related mental health disciplines. The explosion of art therapy education and the organization of a national professional association will be discussed further in the next chapter.

Notes:

[1] For example, Mary Huntoon became an art therapist at the Menninger Foundation in Topeka, Kansas, in 1935.

[2] In addition to regular lectures on the East Coast, Naumburg taught at New York University, the New School for Social Research, presented at annual

meetings of the American Orthopsychiatric Association, the American Psychiatric Association, and the American Psychological Association, and traveled to such places as California, Hawaii, and Texas. (See early issues of the *Bulletin of Art Therapy*.)

3 Much of the personal information about Margaret Naumburg's life comes from the recollections of her son, Thomas Frank (see Detre et al., 1983).

4 The six case studies in this book had been published separately (see Naumburg, 1943, 1944a, 1944b, 1945a, 1945b, & 1946). A revised edition was published as *An Introduction to Art Therapy* (Naumburg, 1973).

5 Tributes to Margaret Naumburg were published in *Art Therapy: Journal of the American Art Therapy Association*, Volume 1, No. 1, 1983, and the *American Journal of Art Therapy*, Volume 22, No. 4, 1983.

6 Menninger himself was a painter and in his later years spent time at the easel until his death in 1990.

7 Lyle later married Karl Menninger (Friedman, 1990, p. 156).

[8] There are some discrepancies as to exactly when Huntoon worked at the Menninger Foundation and Clinic. See Hagaman (1986, p. 25) and Jones (1983, p. 24-25).

[9] This letter and the other figures in this chapter and Chapter Three come from the AATA Archives. None of the typographical errors or sexist language has been changed.

[10] Art by Adamson's patients was used by E. Cunningham Dax in his book *Experimental Studies in Psychiatric Art* (1953).

[11] For accounts of British art therapy from an American viewpoint see Betensky (1971) and Ulman and Champernowne (1963).

[12] This was a bimonthly report on the research project. It also contained case studies and other articles related to art therapy. It ceased publication when the grant ended.

[13] Levy's contributions to art therapy are represented in a memorial issue of the *American Journal of Art Therapy*, Volume 23, No. 2, 1984.

14 More on disputes over AJAT can be found in the *AATA Newsletter,* Volume 13, No. 2, April, 1983.

15 For additional details on Ulman's life and contributions see the *American Journal of Art Therapy*, Volume 30, No. 3, 1992 (a memorial issue with an obituary, tributes, and reprints of her major articles and editorials) and *Art Therapy: Journal of the American Art Therapy Association*, Volume 9, No. 1, 1992.

16 See Chapter 3 for further discussion of this issue. For comparison, the Appendix contains Ulman's minutes of the 1969 meeting.

17 A footnote in Kwiatkowska (1978, p. 86) states "a free picture is one for which no subject is assigned; the patient and his family may draw whatever they wish."

18 This was based on Florence Cane's (1951) technique. However, Elkisch (1948) seems to have been the first to publish on its therapeutic application.

19 Kwiatkowska's obituary appeared in the *American Journal of Art Therapy, 18*: 118–119.

20 The "canes and crutches" refer to Kwiatkowska's orthopedic problems which plagued her for decades. Her experience with hospital treatment made her eager to extend art therapy to medical patients, especially those on orthopedic units (Gantt, 1991, personal communication).

21 Kagin now uses her maiden name Graves.

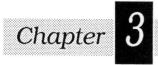

Chapter 3

Expansion
&
Consolidation

The next period in the history of art therapy was one of immense growth and innovation, of expansion and consolidation. By the end of the 1960s, a national professional organization for art therapists, the American Art Therapy Association (AATA), was formed. It provided a forum for communication and debate, and signaled the beginning of art therapy as an organized mental health profession. AATA initiated yearly conferences to bring art therapists from all over the country to share their work with each other and with interested mental health professionals. Standards for a national professional registration (signified by the letters "A.T.R." and standing for "Art Therapist, Registered")[1] were established by AATA along with guidelines for art therapy education. Training programs multiplied. By the mid-1970s, AATA's Education and Training Board began to grant the status of "Approved" to those programs meeting its specific educational requirements. This was an effort to insure quality control, enhance the further development of the field, and safeguard its future.

In the 1970s, a new theoretical position for art therapy grew out of the human potential movement. A small group of art therapists emerged using Jungian psychology and concepts and practitioners began to report case studies in which art therapy was the primary, rather than adjunctive, treatment. Art therapy literature in both article and book form flourished and by the mid-1980s there were three journals in the field: *Art Therapy: Journal of the American Art Therapy Association, The American Journal of Art Therapy,* and *The Arts in Psychotherapy.*

Many of the first art therapists had practiced in psychiatric hospitals or came out of art education as art teachers. This period was one of expanding employment of art therapists in all kinds of facilities and with a wide variety of populations. The years from the 1960s through the mid-1970s were ones of expansion and optimism in mental health. The development of the major tranquilizers and President John F. Kennedy's creation of community mental health centers[2] brought long-term mental patients out of the back wards of hospitals to be treated in their home communities. With de-institutionalization, art therapists began to work in outpatient community mental health clinics, crisis units, pain and stress programs, day treatment hospital programs for the chronically ill, therapeutic and public schools, residential treatment centers, private practice, with the physically disabled, at drug and alcohol facilities, and with clients of all ages. Art therapists extended their practice to work not only with individuals and groups, but also with couples and families.

Also in the 1980s, with increased recognition of the problem of physical and sexual abuse, mental health practitioners, lawyers, and judges examined the artwork of children for possible indicators of abuse (Wohl & Kaufman, 1985; Malchiodi, 1990). Whereas previously, most art therapists had worked under the direction of a psychiatrist or as adjunctive to another therapist, by the mid-1970s, some training programs educated art therapists to function as primary therapists carrying major responsibility for case management, assessment and diagnosis, and treatment. Even for those clients not necessarily interested in or competent in art, the value of art therapy was recognized. Increasingly, the mental health professions acknowledged it as a unique communicative tool that could provide important explicit and implicit information about a client's typical behavior as exhibited in the art task and process as well as a window into the inner life through imagery.

In 1963, Elinor Ulman found only 30 art therapists in the United States and Canada.

> Just as I was starting the *Bulletin*, I sent around a "snowball" questionnaire, trying to locate art therapists.... I found 30 people who called themselves art therapists or thought they might be. A substantial majority of these had a clinical orientation, that is, they viewed patient art as "symbolic speech" and said that a therapeutic endeavor in which art served this function was an important goal of their practice. However, many of these therapists believed that providing adequate conditions for the creative process was likewise important. (Ulman in Jordan, 1988, p. 108)

Over 30 years later, the American Art Therapy Association has a membership of more than 4000.

The Reagan-Bush years (1980–1992) brought severe budget cuts in mental health, the reorganization and limitation of services, and a reassessment of the efficacy of psychotherapy in general. Many chronic patients, released into communities without the necessary services to help them, constituted an increasing percentage of the homeless population in America. Nonetheless, in the 1980s, organized art therapy made gains into the public consciousness and was included in federal regulations[3] for the first time. Increasingly known to the general public, art therapy took its place beside the other mental health professions.

FORMATION OF THE AMERICAN ART THERAPY ASSOCIATION

By the mid-1960s, the formation of a professional organization for art therapists was an idea whose time had come. In the early 1960s, Don Jones and Robert Ault, a young art therapist from Texas, were working at the Menninger Clinic, dreaming together over endless cups of coffee about a national society. As early as 1966, art therapists attended the meeting of the International Society of Psychopathology of Expression in Washington, DC, and talked about forming a group. These art therapists included Sandra Kagin,[4] then living in Oklahoma and working with retarded children; Marge Howard, also from Oklahoma, who had worked in mental health for some years and had done studies on sexually abused children and their artwork; Elinor Ulman; and Tarmo Pasto.

The International Society of Psychopathology of Expression focused its scholarly interests on the pathology evident in artwork. It had been formed in 1959 and included a wide variety of disciplines related to psychopathology and psychology of the arts, although it tended to be dominated by psychiatrists. The American Society had been incorporated in 1966 in Topeka, Kansas. Some of the conference papers from these two groups were published in books edited by Irene Jakab (Jakab 1971, 1969, 1968).

The art therapists, who talked together about the possibility of their own group, envisioned an organization that would be responsive to their needs and would address questions of treatment as well as pathology and diagnosis. However, it is clear from reading the tables of contents of Jakab's publications that art therapists were regular presenters and involved participants. An early volume (Jakab, 1969) includes papers by Margaret Howard, Elsie Muller, Bernard Stone, Donald Uhlin, Tarmo Pasto, and Harriet Wadeson. At one time or another, Pasto, Howard, and Muller were officers in the Society. All became active in the new professional organization for art therapists.

One must wonder why the need for a separate organization was felt so strongly. The 1960s in America was an era of tremendous civil rights activity led by Dr. Martin Luther King, Jr. It may be speculated that in an organization such as the International Society of Psychopathology of Expression dominated by psychiatrists and in a mental health community still hierarchical and based on the medical model, art therapists had the political foresight to recognize that in order to achieve acknowledgement as respected mental health professionals, they would have to separate themselves out. They needed to band together to set up principles of practice and, most essentially, to establish a sense of professional identity. This kind of separatism of a minority group is sometimes an unwanted result of prejudice, but is also a much-practiced strategy and a recognizable first step of minority groups of all kinds to achieve equality.

Don Jones described the Society as having something of a "caste system" in which the art therapists were "invited guests." The art therapists wanted to talk about using the art as treatment, rather than just a measure of pathology, and this was a reason for another organization (Jones, 1993, personal communication).

When Margaret Naumburg's book *Dynamically Oriented Art Therapy* was published in 1966, it provided an important impetus to the new movement. In it, she formally defined the theoretical assumptions that had been presented in her previous books and which she had discussed in presentations throughout the country. In May, 1968, a group of East Coast art therapists[5] coincidentally exhibited artwork of hospitalized psychiatric patients at the meetings of the American Psychiatric Association (APA) in Boston[6] (Figure 3). Later, a panel was presented on art therapy, organized and moderated by Mardi J. Horowitz, MD, at the American Psychiatric Association meetings in Miami Beach. Naumburg, Ulman, Kramer, Kwiatkowska, Carolyn Kniazzeh,[7] and Myra Levick made presentations which were discussed by Paul Jay Fink, MD, and Lyman C. Wynne, MD. This event proved to be extremely significant. Levick writes:

> The separate exhibits were impressive, professional and reflected different approaches within a relatively new modality for the diagnosis and treatment of mentally ill populations—art therapy.... During this conference we were all invited to lunch by Paul J. Fink, M.D., then coordinator of Education and Training at Hahnemann Medical College, now Hahnemann University.... Over lunch we agreed that in order to define this discipline as a recognized profession, a national art therapy association needed to be established. (Levick, 1985, p. 28)

Several Art Therapists, all exhibiting aspects of Art Therapy at The Conventional of The American Psychiatric Association in Boston, May 12-17, 1968, met to discuss the possibility of establishing an American Society of Art Therapists.

Those attending were: Miss Margaret Naumburg - N.Y., N.Y.
                              Mrs. Jane Gilbert - Boston Mass.
                              Miss Lynn Berger, New York, N.Y.
                              Miss Carolyn Refsness - Boston, Mass.
                              Mrs. Hanna Kwiatowska - Bethesda, Md.
                              Miss Miriam Dergalis - Boston, Mass.
                              Mrs. Myra Levick - Philadelphia, Pa.

Also attending were: Mardi Horowitz, M.D. - U.C. Medical
                              School - San Francisco, Calif.

                              Paul Jay Fink, M.D. - Hahnemann
                              Hospital & Medical College -
                              Philadelphia, Pennsylvania

Questions were raised regarding members and officers of the proposed organization and complications that might arise due to the variety of background and training. Dr. Fink explained the "grandfather clause" which is applied to those members beginning any new organization and precedes the establishment of criteria for future members. All those art therapists who are and have been actively engaged in our profession will be invited to become charter members of the organization under this clause. Eventually this organization could serve as the certifying agency for art therapists across the nation. It could also serve to develop art therapists as recognized ancillary personnel in governmental agencies and hospitals.

Miss Naumburg raised the question of funds for establishment and running the association and the need for support form psychiatrists. Dr. Fink voiced the need for art therapist to establish themselves professionally with psychiatrists as consultants. Mrs. Kwiatowska also urged the use of consultant psychiatrists to aid in establishing new programs.

Dr. Horowiz suggested we plan a panel for the next A.P.A. meeting consisting of four papers presented by art therapist and discussed by psychoanalysts. Some tentative suggestions were: "Group Art Therapy," by Lynn Berger; Theoretical Considerations based on Case Material - "What Images Do In Therapy" by Carolyn

Refsness; "Family painting as a Research Technique" by Hanna Kwiatowska; "Art - As part of Milieu Therapy" by Myra Levick. Dr. Horowitz suggested we send ideas to him and he would submit them to the A.P.A. The deadline to the A.P.A. is September 20.

Dr, Fink and Dr. Horowitz offered to discuss papers and other names such as Dr. Norman Brattle, Mass., Dr. Selroh of Boston and Dr. William Niederland of New York were also proposed as possible participants. Mrs. Kwiatowska said she would discuss the possibility of sponsorship for this program with her superiors at N.I.M.H. Bethesda, Maryland. Since the deadline is very soon for submitting an application based on the above, and the details sent to the A.P.A. later.

Those present agreed the establishment of such an organization would do much to help establish Art Therapy as an important ancillary psychiatric modality, but evaluations, standard and goals must be clarified.

Myra Levick offered to send copies of the minutes to those present and other names suggested with request for individual ideas on the proposals stated to be sent to her. Mrs. Levick also said she would try to plan a meeting for these people to come together to discuss these ideas sometime in the fall.

Respectfully submitted,

(Mrs.) Myra F. Levick, M.Ed.
Acting Secretary

Figure 3 (cont.)

The First Organizational Meeting

The first formal attempt to form a national organization for art therapists took place in 1968, under the auspices of Hahnemann Hospital in Philadelphia. Dr. Fink was tremendously interested in art therapy and he, along with Morris Goldman, MD, Director of Hahnemann's Community Mental Health Center, had begun what was the first graduate-level art therapy training program (called "Psychiatric Art Therapy") since the program in the 1950s at Louisville had become inactive. Myra Levick was hired as Director. In 1967, Levick, Fink, and Goldman had published an article in the *Bulletin of Art Therapy* called "Training for Art Therapists." Elinor Ulman acknowledged Levick as "the founding spirit of the association" (Ulman in Jordan, 1988, p. 108).

Levick had attended Moore College of Art in Philadelphia and later earned her doctorate from Bryn Mawr College:

> I was trained as a professional artist—having gone back to school after marriage and children...I have painted all my life.... At the time I graduated Moore College, I had been considering going on for a Master's degree in the History of Art. In fact I had been accepted and there was a little notice on the bulletin board that a psychiatrist was look-

ing for an artist to work with emotionally disturbed patients in the first inpatient unit in a general hospital in
Philadelphia. I was absolutely fascinated. He said that he
thought an artist had a great deal to offer in working with
emotionally disturbed patients and if I would bring my art
skills, he would teach me how. He told me there were art
therapists in the country about which I knew nothing. I
gave up the History of Art Master's and he took me on.
(Levick, 1975a)

So, in 1963, she:

had the opportunity to utilize my talent and training as a
painter in a 29-bed inpatient unit for adults suffering from
moderate neurosis to severe psychosis...my job title was
"art therapist" and one of my first tasks was to learn what
that implied. (Levick, 1983a, p. 11)

Although many had talked of the need for a national
association, it was Myra Levick's energy (along with
Paul Fink's encouragement) which brought about the
necessary steps to create the organization. Levick's role
in the formation of the American Art Therapy Association irrevocably changed the course of art therapy in the
United States by emphasizing art therapy as a separate
discipline (as had been defined by Naumburg) and
thereby fostering the emerging sense of identity of the art
therapist as a special kind of mental health practitioner.
Levick was the American Art Therapy Association's first

president[7] and has been actively involved with its progress since then. She eventually became Director of the Creative Arts in Therapy Program at Hahnemann which included dance and music therapies as well. She published widely and became the editor of the second journal in the field, *The Arts in Psychotherapy* (originally called *Art Psychotherapy*). In 1983, Levick published *They Could Not Talk and So They Drew*, which dealt with defense mechanisms as they were expressed in art. Levick wrote: "My own particular interest and expertise evolved around ego mechanisms of defense...how these elements are manifested in drawings of children and adults in a therapeutic milieu" (Levick, 1983a, p. xviii). She is now retired and living in Florida while continuing to consult as an art therapist.

In December 1968, Myra Levick and Paul Fink hosted an organizational meeting (Figures 4–7) and invited as many art therapists as they could find.[9] About 85 people (including 50 art therapists) attended, and an *ad hoc* steering committee was elected. The committee consisted of Elinor Ulman, Don Jones, Felice Cohen, Robert Ault, and Myra Levick. (Robert Ault was hired by Don Jones at the Menninger Foundation in 1960 and had been trained by Jones.) The steering committee was given the task of developing a constitution for the new organization.

From the beginning, there was considerable and sometimes acrimonious controversy over whether to form an organization at all. Although many art therapists saw the need for a forum to bring people together for the purposes of education and identity and to achieve recognition as a new profession, a few, such as Elinor Ulman felt that it was too soon and that art therapy should develop further on its own.[10] She and Edith Kramer urged that a broader territory be carved out for the field, one which went beyond psychiatric settings (Figure 8).

While some were trying to slow what they felt to be a premature definition of the field, others were convinced that forming a national association was urgent. Don Jones remembers he went

> with a sense of frustration. Having written to art therapy people and others saying we must get together...at that time my impression from them was that we can't form an organization. This is a very special kind of thing. It can only be taught by selected practitioners. Myra...told me her impression of my coming to Philadelphia which was: I walked into her office, thumped my fist on her table...and said either we get it together *now* or forget it! I felt the urgent need. If we were going to grow at all we needed to get together. (Jones, 1975)

THE HAHNEMANN MEDICAL COLLEGE AND HOSPITAL OF PHILADELPHIA

230 North Broad Street   Philadelphia, Pa.   19102

TO: Art Therapists

FROM: Myra Levick, M.Ed.
           Director of Art Therapy
           Hahnemann Community Mental Health Center

SUBJECT: Formation of the American Society of Art Therapists

****

        In an earlier communication you received a copy of the minutes of
a meeting which took place in Boston, May, 1968.

        In those minutes a meeting was suggested for sometime in the win-
ter in conjunction with one of the guest lecture series held here at
Hahnemann Medical College. The schedule for the guest lecture series is
enclosed.

        On December 5, 1968 Miss Elinor Ulman will be our guest speaker.
At that time we would like to invite you to attend a pre-lecture meeting
at the college from 2:30 to 4:00 p.m. for the purpose of getting acquainted
over coffee and cake and discussing the formulation of a national organization. Following the lecture we will have cocktails and hors d' oeuvres.

        As our list of practicing art therapists is far from complete, we
hope you will extend this invitation to any art therapists in your community who would be interested and able to attend.

        We would greatly appreciate a reply by November 15, 1968 so that we
may know how many people to prepare for.

        We sincerely hope you can attend, but if this is not possible, we
would like to know your feelings and suggestions regarding this proposal
so that we may communicate them to those present.

Figure 4

A G E N D A

For December 5, 1968 Meeting

2:30 p.m. to 3:00 p.m.

1. Greetings from Mrs. M. Levick, V.O. Hammett, M.D., and Paul Jay Fink, M.D.

   Introduction of Art Therapy Faculty

3:00 p.m. - on

2. Purpose of meeting - to formulate national organization of art therapists

   Discussion, motion, and vote

3. Criteria for training of art therapists - Dr. Paul Jay Fink

   Discussion

4. Report on proposed panel at A.P.A. Meeting in May in Florida   -   Dr. Mardi Horowitz

5. Vote for temporary officers

6. Selection of following committees by those present

   (1) Nomination
   (2) Credentials
   (3) Training criteria
   (4) Bylaws

7. Plans for next meeting - Mr. Robert Ault, Menninger Clinic

Figure 5

Minutes For Art Therapy Meeting
HELD IN PHILADELPHIA ON
December 5, 1968

****

The meeting was attended by approximately eighty people from all over the country. Fifty of these people were art therapists, the other thirty consisted of psychiatrists, educators, etc. It was decided that only art therapists would vote on any motions.

Greetings from Mrs. Levick, V.O. Hammett, M.D., and Paul Jay Fink, M.D. Mrs. Levick introduced the art therapy faculty - those introduced were: Dr. Bodarky, Executive Director, Hahnemann Community Mental Health Center, Dr. Vaccaro, Dr. Nathan, Dr. Weinburg, Dr. Wolfe, Dr. Goldman, and E. Gentner.

Mrs. Levick then proceeded to the next point on the agenda which was the purpose of the meeting: to form a National Organization of Art Therapists.

Dr. Fink presented the criterion for training art therapists here at Hahnemann. A discussion followed:

Mr. Ault made one point: at Menninger, art therapists may be doing all kinds of things, not just art therapy. They must have a broader definition of the work. Mr. Metzler, from Baltimore, questioned if these students are artists. Dr. Fink replied that they are graduates of art colleges.

Dr. Speck addressed himself to Dr. Fink and asked, "as relates to teaching and education, you (Dr. Fink) strongly emphasized clinical experience; where does this leave room for well trained educators?" Dr. Fink replied by stating that we here have gotten students into the Board of Education to conduct classes. The variety of programs in going to be as great as the variety of people who start the program. Dr. Speck felt that one group should not control, and Dr. Fink replied that it's not a matter of control. Dr. Speck then quoted Dr. Fink in his statement on training criterion, in which he (Dr. Fink) stated: "Educators should be utilized in education situations:. Dr. Fink answers by stating that you might want your students to have a more basic understanding of education principles. Dr. Speck stated that medical art therapist should be supervised by a medical person, psychiatric art therapists by a psychiatrist, etc., and questioned if these people are specially trained in art therapy. Mrs. Levick pointed out that students rotate through public schools. "Mrs. Schoenfelder, director, is here", she continued, "and we supervise students in connection with classroom situations. We have coordinated throughout students' experiences. The director of schools is directly involved, and we communicate with each other as much as possible."

Figure 6

Dr. Fink then emphasized that it is a matter of multiple supervision; that if only one supervisor is available, that the supervisor should be an art therapist. Miss Naumburg said that she sees this as psychiatrists still being in control.

Dr. White, who is the Clinical Director of Norton Clinic, in Louisville, Kentucky, expressed his view that in setting up the program, "as to who should be parent - medical school should not; educational school should not either; nor should the Department of Fine Arts. Others involved in supervising the program tend to dominate the field, and I am no exception. It is very important in establishing this - I would advise the group that it should be a multiple faceted program. It would be a mistake otherwise, a disservice to the organization."

Dr. Vaccaro said that in approaching the question philosophically, "We have to understand the object of what we are doing. It is our understanding that whenever someone communicates material distressing, it is a form of communication and expression (suffering) in him, and because of this we act therapeutically, if not we have no place in psychiatry. Philosophically, it is not a question of control (psychiatry, education). What is a person trying to do by communication by means of nonverbal communication? If not therapy, it is nothing. What does the person need who is committed to your care? Educators are concerned with training the student, as a doctor is with treating conflict. I think most is the care of the person be placed in the hands of the Mental Health Center. What we are trying to do is to assimilate unifying concepts of the whole person from discipline of education, health, psychiatry, in order to understand what people are trying to communicate to us through this nonverbal means of artistic expression."

Dr. Franz brought out that it is not a matter of whether it is supervision by psychiatrists; it obvious that we would bring psychiatrists into it. When looking at criterion of training for art therapy, it seems to minimize that art therapy is a unique technique of its own and has an integrity of its own. He went on to say that supervision with psychiatrists is part of it; training as an art therapist is primary. Art therapy has techniques of its own different from verbal psychotherapy.

Dr. Fink explained that his concept of the meeting was for the art therapists to set up an organization for themselves. He did not think that psychiatrists should be members, and stated that the organization was set up and handled by art therapists.

Miss Ulman then emphasized that if art therapy divorced itself from art, it has lost its purpose of being. Miss Naumburg stated that she didn't feel that the group was considering that, and added, "You talk about it as though art therapy was just beginning as a modality". Mrs. Levick pointed out that if the group did not recognize all that has been accomplished by art therapists in the past, it would not meeting to establish this as a recognized profession. Miss Naumburg replied that it would not be the same because it would be controlled by psychiatrists, analysts, etc. She felt that the group

Figure 6 (cont.)

was not ready yet. Mrs. Levick argued that the people were there because they wanted to get together to set up this organization. Mr. Ault went on to say, "The reason people are her today is because we have been working independently throughout the country. The purpose is to accumulate knowledge through this organization. I want to increase my understanding of what art therapy is about. Mrs. Cohen brought out that she did not feel anyone was arguing art as art therapy, but art or therapy. She then mentioned Virginia Austin's letter to the group, and said that this reflected her own thinking, also.

Claire Sherr brought up a question about the list of criterion, and said that it seemed to be a double standard, in that it takes 10 years to learn any one of the subjects well and the students are to learn them in 10 months.

Mr. Jones said that this has to be a loose organization until consolidated:
1.   Our relationship with art therapy
2.   Our organization with magazines, National Art Education Association might profit by relating self.
3.   Relating to one another through news letters, etc.

Because of the time elements Mrs. Levick ended the discussion and went of to the next point, which was an invitation from Bob Ault to have the next meeting in the spring at the Menninger Clinic in Topka, Kansas. Mr. Jones motioned to set up a temporary structure for the organization of an Art Therapy Association. Mr. Anthony then seconded the motion.

Miss Naumburg then brought up financial problems involved with mailing, etc. Miss Ulman suggested communications be established and a collection of information in addition to the Data Sheet Mrs. Levick said had been given out to everyone at the meeting. Mr. Metzler pointed out that since everyone here was involved in differint situations, they should submit a short paragraph on their program, its functions, and relation to psychiatry.

Mrs. Cohen then made the motion that we elect Mrs. Levick as a temporary president of the organization, and Mr. Metzler seconded the motion. Miss Ulman said that she thought that Miss Naumburg should be entrusted with this, and Mr. Ault then brought up the fact that the motion to set up an organization had not been voted on yet. Mrs. Levick called for a vote and the motion was carried. Mr. Ault then suggested nominations for a committee, and Dr. Fink seconded the motion. It was voted on as yes.

Harriet Wadeson suggested that the committee be limited to people representing various areas of the country, such as New York, Philadelphia, Washington, D.C. etc. Mr. Taylor said this should be something for committee members to decide, as to whether or not they are willing to travel distances to communicate with each other.

Miss Naumburg then suggested some amount of dues from everyone present for future funds for mailing be requested.

Figure 6 (cont.)

Dr. White listed some suggestions for the Steering Committee: that they should propose constitution and by-laws, establish what the organization is all about, and suggest appropriate dues. He said that the committee structure should be of those who are interested in sitting down with and making up policies, constitution, by-laws, etc. He stated that until we establish that, we are not ready to go into criterion for training.

The vote was taken for five of the seven nominees for the Steering Committee, and the seven nominations were:

M. Naumburg	F. Cohen
D. Jones	R. Ault
M. Levick	E. Kramer
E. Ulman	

Those elected by vote were:

M. Levick	F. Cohen
D. Jones	R. Ault
E. Ulman	

Mr. Brown then motioned that this committee be an ad hoc committee that would be appointed to investigate the needs for development of such an organization.

Mrs. Levick called for suggestions for date for the next meeting. Mr. Ault said that the facilities at the Menninger Clinic would be available and they would be willing to host sometime in the spring. he said that it would be available any time except for one date, April 25th. Dr. Roger White also offered the Norton Mental Health Center in Louisville, Kentucky as another possible location. Mr. Jones suggested that the Steering Committee nominate a meeting place.

the meeting was then adjourned.

Respectfully submitted, Ann O'kane, acting secretary.

MEMO

TO -   Dr. Harding, Dr. George, Mr. Hanson

FROM -   Don Jones

SUBJECT -   Report on the Art Therapy Seminar December 5, 1968

On December 5 a group of eighty people met at the Hahneman Hospital and Medical College in Philadelphia for the purpose of exploring the forming of an American Association of Art Therapists. Although the group was made up predominately of practicing art therapy people from various parts of the country, there were a number of psychiatrists, psychologists and educators present. The creation of a national organization for art therapists is not a new idea. Many dedicated people working in isolated situations throughout the country, as a matter of fact, throughout the world, have hoped to accomplish this goal. Such an organization is essential to further the development of training programs; to standardize criteria for training and development of therapeutic techniques; and to facilitate the communication among the various art therapists in the discipline of psychiatry. Ultimately, such an organization could serve as a certifying agency for art therapists throughout the country.

I was pleased to have the opportunity to attend this meeting because of my personal interest and efforts over the years in art therapy and in the formation of such a national organization. To me, it seemed that the meeting was a success from the start. It was the first time that such a large group of art therapists from across the country had ever gotten together. The group did take some concrete steps in forming an organization. The spirit of the group from the outset was one of seriousness of purpose and desire to accomplish something.

In subsequent meetings we discussed the criteria for training of art therapists. We reviewed in brief some of the various philosophical approaches to the use of art therapy and its' application as a treatment tool in psychiatry, rehabilitation, and education. The discussion was rich and the views ranged from that of the art teacher to that of the psychoanalytical-oriented therapist using art.

The final work of the conference was to elect a temporary steering committee and to charge it with the responsibility of designing the initial administrative machinery of the organization. Five people representing different parts of the country will be serving on this committee. They include Mr. Robert Ault, of the Menninger Hospital, Topeka, Kansas, Mrs. Felice Cohen of the Child Guidance Center of Houston, Texas, Don Jones of the Harding Hospital, Worthington, Ohio, Mrs. Myra Levich of the Hahneman Community Mental Health Center in Philadelphia, and Mrs. Elinor Ulman, consultant in art therapy to the Northern Virginia Mental Health Institute. This group will begin to collect data from all those who are practicing art therapy in different parts of the United States and Canada. They will also begin some systematic publicity to medical

Figure 7

journals and psychiatric institutions informing them of the Philadelphia meeting and the intention of the group to form a national art therapy organization. In the process they will be enlisting the support of various psychiatrists who have shown an interest in art therapy.

I feel that this had been an important first step. I recommend that we at Harding Hospital lend our interest and support.

Don Jones

DLJ:fc

Dear Bob –
Here is a copy of my initial report to the hospital here. Tho't you might be interested.
I have been doing a little surveying here in Columbus and have found quite a group in practice + at the university. We are going to get together soon.
I was delighted to have "extra" time to tour the gallery and renew our friendship. I was pleased that you seemed happy and confident.

Best Regards
Don

SUGGESTIONS CONCERNING AN AMERICAN ASSOCIATION OF ART THERAPISTS

By Edith Kramer, Supervisor of Art Therapy, Albert Einstein College of
Medicine; Art Therapist, Jewish Guild for the Blind;
Consultant in Art Therapy, Hahnemann Medical College;
Member of the Faculty, New School for Sxa Social
Research and Turtle Bay Music School.

and Elinor Ulman, Editor, Bulletin of Art Therapy; Consultant in Art
Therapy, Northern Virginia Mental Health Institute;
Member of the Faculty, Washington School of Psychiatry;
Assistant Professorial Lecturer, The George Washington
University.

(These Comments are being sent to all art therapists and physicians who were
present at the Boston meeting of May 14, 1968 concerned with the formation of
an association of art therapists.)

We are aware of the need for a national association of art therapists and
iax in sympathy with the intentions implied in the Minutes of the Boston
meeting of May 14, 1968 and the Objectives and Philosophy prepared by Myra
Levick in consultation with her psychiatric colleagues at Hahnemann Medical
College. We are writing to suggest only that such an association should from
the staxi beginning seek a broader base than that defined or assumed in those
documents.

Art therapy has already proved itself not only in mental hospitals and
other institutions directed by psychiatrists, but also in many settings where
psychiatric supervision or consultation is scarce or altogether lacking.
Examples may be found in special schools and classes for the retarded, the
delinquent, the deaf, and the blind; in homes for the aged, and neighborhood
houses, and prisons--in sum, wherever the rehabilitation of the physically,
emotionally, mentally, or socially handicapped is a seriously undertaken. The
well-trained art therapist must, therefore, be prepared to act both
judiciously and independently out of a highly developed understanding of his
own field.

It goes without saying that the philosophy of art therapy and the
training to be developed for the profession must take into account insights
derived from psychiatry and psychoanalysis. Some art therapists can be
expected, in the future as at present, to serve in psychiatric instituions
in an ancillary capacity. We feel, however, that the sense of the Boston
meeting as reported in the Minutes, which state that an organization of art
therapists "would do much to help establish Art Therapy as an important
ancillary psychiatric modality," and of the Objectives and Philosophy which
calls for sharing "thoughts and experiences...within the discipline of
psychiatry" needs to be carefully reconsidered.

The future of art therapy will be much brighter if those who formulate the
objectives of the first national organization of art therapists look to
an independent place in the broad field of sxaia special education and
rehabilitation rather than ixxxixy limiting their sphere to that of an
ancillary psychiatric discipline.

September 19, 1968

Figure 8   103

Of the meeting in Philadelphia, Robert Ault says:

> Don Jones and I spent years working together and sitting
> in a back room drinking coffee and talking about someday
> maybe creating a national organization. We had dreamed
> about that and shared [that dream] for a long time.... Don
> left Menninger's very shortly before the first meeting. If
> Don had still been at Menninger's, one of us would have
> had to stay home to cover at the hospital. As it was, we
> both went to Philadelphia to work on a project that we
> had both wanted as our big life project. (Ault, 1975)

Ault continues about the Philadelphia meeting:

> [That first meeting was] very heated. Margaret Naumburg
> was there. She was a very old woman with a hearing loss.
> She would sit with her cane and every time someone said
> something she didn't want to hear, she would knock her
> cane on the floor. She was nominated [to the steering
> committee] but lost and stomped out saying "I'm not
> through with you!" I had several warm pleasant letters
> from her later but those initial days, they were something
> else! (Ault, 1975)

Rawley Silver from New Rochelle, New York, attended the Philadelphia organizing meeting; her feeling
about it was shared by a number of others. "As someone
working in an isolated situation," she said, "I was delighted to meet others who shared my interests and concerns" (Silver, 1985).

The steering committee worked for several months (Figures 9–12) and then set up a meeting at the University of Louisville, Kentucky, on June 27, 1969. Naumburg was unable to attend (Figure 13) and there were several disagreements on key issues. There were opposing opinions on the form the association should take. In Washington, Ulman worked on a constitution for the new organization, while in Kansas, Robert Ault consulted with Bill Sears of the Music Therapy Department at University of Kansas. In 1954, Sears had helped create the National Association for Music Therapy. Ault also collected constitutions from the American Speech and Hearing Association, the American Occupational Therapy Association, and the Wisconsin Art Therapy Association, a state art therapy organization. He concluded the best structure was one which

> emphasiz[ed] a strong federal organization with the possibility of eventual state or local chapters or units. The day before attending the committee meeting in Louisville, I drafted a constitution and had copies made to take along. As it turned out, Elinor had also brought copies of a constitutional model she had put together...that of a rather weak national alliance composed of strong state units. The discussions of the committee were long and difficult, ending at 4 a.m. The next day a constitution was read to the assembled group and adopted (Ault, 1975).

The First Executive Board

Having adopted a constitution[11] based on the model of a strong national body, the members of the new organization elected officers and committee chairs: Myra Levick, President; Robert Ault, President-Elect; Margaret Howard (Oklahoma), Treasurer; Felice Cohen (Texas), Secretary; Elsie Muller (Missouri), Constitution; Sandra Kagin (Kentucky), Education; Helen Landgarten (California), Public Information; Don Jones (Ohio), Publications; Ben Ploger (Louisiana), Professional Standards; Bernard Stone (Ohio), Membership; and Hanna Yaxa Kwiatkowska (Washington, DC), Research.

Many on the original Executive Board such as Levick, Kagin, and Landgarten went on to contribute to the field as authors and/or as directors of training programs. Their other accomplishments will be discussed in the next chapter. However, in an evolving clinical discipline it is natural that many would put their primary energies into clinical work. Ben Ploger had begun teaching art in Houston in 1935. He became professor and chair of the Department of Fine Arts at Delgado College in New Orleans. There, according to Levick, he was asked to "volunteer time to teach art to mentally disturbed nuns

April 16, 1969

Miss. Elinor Ulman,
1789 Lanier Place, N.W.,
Apartment 23,
Washington, D.C.   20009

Dear Miss. Ulman:

I want you to know how pleased I am that you have decided
to continue working with the committee. There can be no
doubt that because of this decision, our committee is greatly
enhanced and the realization of an American Society of Art
Therapists is closer to becoming a reality.

You were correct when you suggested that I was not in a
calm mood when I wrote the letter to which you referred.
I believe that the need is so great for the formation of a
national society and I also believe that your years of
experience, knowledge, integrity and support are of importance
in furthering this aim. In your correspondence, which
predicated my letter in question, it seemed to me that you
implied that the viewpoints of some of the members of the
committee were irresponsible and not qualified-- this I found
difficult to accept and my mood was definitely affected.

I want us to be a cohesive group with a positive goal and
since it would appear that you feel that my letter which you
received March 7, 1969 contained distortions, I feel compelled
to give you the facts I do have and perhaps the air can be
cleared. I am not writing this for the purpose of soliciting
further explanation or to continue on with this subject
matter but only in the hope that you will appreciate that I,
like you, also had reactions to this situation and such
reactions were derived from the relevant facts I have on
hand. After reading your letter of April 1, 1969, I am
better able to understand how and why you do feel as you do.
It is my hope that after you have read this letter, you will
understand how and why I reacted the way I did.

The omission of a date on the letter was simply an error on
my part. As I stated, my typing leaves much to be desired
and this error of omission was just one of many typographical
errors in the letter.

Figure 9

There can be little doubt that I do not have all the relevant facts that you have concerning the Boston meeting, but in deference to both of us, I would like you to know what facts I do have. These facts led me to state that "some 80 individuals besides myself attended the December 5th meeting for the express purpose of founding as American Art Therapy Association.

On June 21, 1968, I received a letter from Dr. Paul Fink in response to my letter inquiring about the training program for art therapists at Hahnemann. A psychiatrist on our staff attended the Boston Meeting and learned of this training program. She suggested that I initiate correspondence for the purpose of gaining information on this subject. In Dr. Fink's letter, he stated that Mrs. Myra Levick was working on "setting up a national organization for art therapists so that training for accredation will be uniform." In a letter from Myra Levick dated July 1, 1968, she referred to attempts being made to set up a national organization for art therapists. She added that, "this idea was conceived by several of us who were exhibiting aspects of art therapy at the Boston Conference." I understood this to mean that the idea was conceived by several art therapists but not that the next or future meetings were to be restricted only to those few art therapists. I am not certain, but I believe that it was at about this time that Myra sent me a mimeographed copy of the minutes of this Boston meeting. In response to all of this, I wrote Myra and offered to be of any help in contacting art therapists in this geographical area and appraising them of the possibility of a meeting to form a national organization.

Subsequently, I received notification of your lecture scheduled for December 5th and of the "founding" meeting to be held just prior to your lecture. Myra wrote that Bob Ault from The Menninger Foundation would be there and this encouraged my notion that interested art therapists from various parts of the country would be at the meeting. Interestingly enough, Before I could inform a dear friend of mine and an art therapists Mrs. Virginia Austin of Houston, of these plans, she called me to say that Miss Naumburg, had written her stating that she, Miss Naumburg, had included Virginia in her attendance list of those whom she wished to notify to invite to the December 5th meeting. I concluded that if Miss. Naumburg invited someone from Houston, Texas to attend, surely others from diversified areas of the country had been invited by others and I again concluded that this would be

a sizable meeting for the purpose of founding a national
organization.

I can appreciate that you anticipated "another small
committee meeting," hopefully you can better understand that
I anticipated a large meeting. Surely, so many would not
have traveled so far and for just a day or so, if they had
not assumed the afore stated plans were to found a national
group.

I am not unaware of the groundwork, leadership, honesty,
integrity and devotion you and "the small, select group worked
to establish in isolation and with little institutuional
support." I am not unmindful that without the years of work
accomplished by these women, art therapy could not have
arrived at the threshold of national recognition that we
now find ourselves. I can only speak for myself so let me
repeat now what I said to you, Miss, Kramer, Mrs. Kwiatkowska,
and Dr. Franz when you all were kind enough to be my guests
for dinner after the December 5th meeting. Art Therapy has
reached the heights it has today as a result of the work all
of you and Miss. Naumburg have contributed. Your names are
synonomous with art therapy. It was a distinct pleasure for
me to sit at a table surrounded by the authors of this
discipline which I have chosen to follow. It is not my
desire to encroach upon the groundwork and devotion of this
small select group but rather to offer what I can to help
establish art therapy as an accepted and recognized discipline
for all qualified art therapists through out this country
through the formation of a national organization for all of us.

I am enclosing a letter anddquestionnaire that is self
explanatory. This is just one of many who are interested
in what our committee is doing. It was not clear in Mrs.
Rubin's letter whether or not she mailed each of you a
copy of this letter and the questionnaire. If she did not,
I felt that each of you would like to have a copy of them.

I regret that I am unable to attend the Miami meeting but
I look forward to the meeting in Louisville in June and I
do agree with Bob Ault that the Steering Committee should
meet the day before the planned meeting.

                          Sincerely,

                          (Mrs.) Felice W. Cohen
                          Art Therapist
enc: 2
cc: Mrs. Myra Levick, Mr. R. Ault, Mr. D. Jones

Figure 9 (cont.)   109

TO WHOM IT MAY CONCERN:

May 8, 1969

We the undersigned, art therapists experienced in work xx in psychiatric and (in some instances) other settings, have read and considered the following documents:

(1) SUGGESTIONS CONCERNING AN AMERICAN ASSOCIATION OF ART THERAPISTS, By Edith Kramer and Elinor Ulman, September 19, 1968

(2) A JOINT STATEMENT FROM: Hanna Yaxa Kwiatkowska, Margaret Naumburg, and Elinor Ulman, November 1968

(3) Letter from Paul Jay Fink, M.D., to Lawrence Kolb, M.D., April 3, 1969

(4) Letter from Elinor Ulman to Paul Jay Fink, M.D., April 24, 1969

(5) PROPOSALS FOR CONSIDERATION AT THE JUNE MEETING, sent by Elinor Ulman to Robert Ault, Felice Cohen, Don Jones, and Myra Levick, April 23, 1969

(6) THE PROBLEM OF NATIONAL ORGANIZATION: MAKE HASTE SLOWLY, by Roy Stern, M.D., and Ethelmary Honoré, Bulletin of Art Therapy, Vol. 8, No. 3, April 1969

As a group we subscribe to the following statements:

"Art therapy has already proved itself not only in mental hospitals and other institutions directed by psychiatrists, but also in many settings where psychiatric supervision or consultation is scarce or altogether lacking....The future of art therapy will be much brighter if those who formulate the objectives of the first national organization of art therapists look to an independent place in the broad field of special education and rehabilitation rather than limiting their sphere to that of an ancillary psychiatric discipline." (1)

"A committee of experienced practicing art therapists should be chosen to consider the range of acceptable approaches to the application of art therapy in psychotherapy, rehabilitation, and education. Suitable types of art therapy training will depend on the definition of these objectives." (2)

We are also concerned with the following issues:

Dr. Fink (3) purported to speak for art therapists and their only elected committee, but not xnxx even the committee members had been consulted by him before his letter was sent (4). Art therapists should exercise their right to formulate their own goals and appoint their own consultants. Dr. Fink's statements are not representative of the opinions expressed by any body of art therapists up to this time.

Dr. Fink's implication that it is time for art therapy to investigate "procedures for the accreditation and the maintaining of training criteria for psychiatric art therapists in the United States" (3) strikes us as premature. These moves should await the development of a number of independent training centers and centers of clinical experimentation, and further development of theory, as Stern and Honoré (6) point out.

Elinor Ulman's tentative formulation of goals and structure for a national federation of art therapy associations (5) should be developed and fully presented at the projected open meeting of art therapists in Louisville, Kentucky, in June 1969. As she stated, this plan will avoid "the pitfalls of rigidity and factionalism so ably expounded by Dr. Stern and Miss Honoré.... When the time for further steps in the direction of nationalization and certification is ripe, the Federation will stand ready, and will be able to take pride in having helped bring such worth-while developments into being."

Those of us who will be unable to attend the June meeting hereby appoint Elinor Ulman as our representative, with full power to vote on our behalf on any matters brought before this meeting.

Carolyn Refsnes Kniazzeh, Art Therapist, Cambridge, Mass.

Edith Kramer, Albert Einstein College of Medicine, N.Y.

Hanna Yaxa Kwiatkowska, Head, Art Therapy Unit, National Institute of Mental Health

Margaret Naumburg, New School for Social Research

Elinor Ulman, Editor, Bulletin of Art Therapy

Figure 10 (cont.)

111

MISS ELINOR ULMAN
APARTMENT 32
1789 LANIER PLACE, N.W.
WASHINGTON, D. C. 20009

June 15, 1969

Dear Fellow Committee Member:

As I wrote on May 20, at an informal meeting on May 9 a majority of th
ad hoc steering committee (Myra Levick, Bob Ault, and I) were "of the opini
that the June 27 agenda should be primarily devoted to dialogue concerning
future organization of art therapists." An undated letter sent on about Ju
10 to the entire mailing list in the name of all members of the committee,
invites participants to present "ideas about the purpose to which they woul
like to see a future organization dedicated and the form they believe such
organization should take." The letter further states that, "An important
purpose of the June 27 meeting will be to put on record a variety of propos
and arguments for wide distribution, so that eventual decisions may be base
on thorough, thoughtful consideration of alternatives and their implicatio

In view of the above, the Resolution sent by Myra Levick on June 11,
proposing that a "national organization for art therapists be erected at
Philadelphia, Pa., on June 27, 1969," and that the accompanying "Statement
Principle and By-Laws serve as the official documents of the organization,"
would, if officially adopted by the ad hoc steering committee of art thera
constitute a clear breach of faith with all who were invited to the June 27
meeting.

As you will see from the enclosed statement dated May 8, 1969, I am
authorized to speak at the Louisville meetings for the five art therapists
originally invited to represent our profession at the 1969 annual meeting o
the American Psychiatric Association. Should a majority of the ad hoc
steering committee adopt the Resolution cited above, it would probably be
necessary to present the May 8 statement and the six supporting documents w
which you are all familiar at the June 27 meeting so as to make them part
of the public record.

I sincerely hope, however, that a majority of the committee will refra
from recommending premature, hasty antiaxxx action at a meeting where ther
can be no possible assurance that those who will be afff affected by decisi
can be adequately represented. I was much cheered by the fact that on May
9 a majority of the ad hoc steering committee realized the importance of
airing all vital issues in an orderly, democratic manner rather than rushin
ahead with decisions that would certainly launch the new organization in an
atmosphere of dissension and bitterness.

The spirit of the May 9 meeting would dictate that the phrase "on June
27, 1969" be stricken from the Resolution. This Resolution would be in orde
as a majority or a minority recommendation for action to be taken after wid
distribution of a variety of proposals and arguments, and by a vote either
conducted through the mail or at a meeting where advance notice was given a
proxy voting invited.

Very sincerely yours,

Elinor Ulman

112   *Figure 11*

June 26, 1969

Dear AD HOC STEERING COMMITTEE and Colleagues:

In response to the letter of request for proposals and arguments concerning the formation of a national federation or society of art therapists, I submit the following points of concern.

I. A definitive outline must be developed of the various roles and duties of all art therapists. Responsibilities and job requirements may differ greatly according to institutions and type of patient material. For instance:

A psychiatric art therapist working with adult psychotics may have a very different experience, training and responsibility than a therapist working only with retarded children.

II. Final definitions or organizational plans must be democratic and broad enough to include all therapist groups. One exclusive model should not serve all situations. For instance:

A psychiatric art therapist, employed by a large state hospital, may not favor or benefit from a role definition that separates the teamwork policy of the art therapist and psychiatrist as contrasted with the independent model favored by some individual workers. Most states do not allow dynamic art psychotherapy to be practiced without medical supervision. Some art therapists, including myself, consider the availability of psychiatric consul, hospital records, and psychologists reports as a professional advantage and not a block to power or progress.

III. I purpose, the future society print a journal or bulletin dedicated to a wide range of ideas and influences concerning art therapy. No one person should edit footnotes, eliminate them and replace them with "chosen persons". There is more than one informed center in the world and such a practice can damage trust and interpersonal relationships. It is delusional to falsely give credit for influences and to attempt to independently direct the course of history.

IV. The proposed society should proceed slowly and by means of democratic process in all major decisions concerning organizational standards, certification, training, and membership.

Respectfully yours,

Bernard O. Stone

Bernard O. Stone
Director, Art Psychotherapy Unit
Columbus State Hospital
Columbus, Ohio

BOS:jes

Figure 12

113

Dear Mr. Ault,

Thank you for your letter inviting me to the University of Louisville meeting concerning the formulation of plans for a National organization of Art Therapists, but I am not able to come at that time

Miss Elinor Ulman will represent my point of view. You probably do not know that in 1956-57 I was invited to the Louisville University + Medical school, to give a number of lectures on Art Therapy. They talked then of wanting me to help them plan an M.A. in Art Therapy for the

University, but they were then totally unprepared to do it at that time

Sincerely,
Margaret Naumburg

P.S I'm enclosing my curriculum Vitae, where you will find and trip to Louisville listed.

M. N.

Figure 13 (cont.)   115

cloistered in the religious unit of the De Paul Hospital"
(Levick, 1981, p. 5). He began to practice art therapy
throughout the hospital and became director of art
psychotherapy there in 1966. Margaret Howard was also
treasurer of the American Society of Psychopathology of
Expression. Having studied with Naumburg, she was
the art therapist at the Children's Medical Center in Tulsa
for many years. Sandra Kagin trained with Howard.
Elsie Muller, a social worker by training, had also
studied with Naumburg; she worked at the Gillis Home
for Children and later the Ozanam Home for Disturbed
Adolescent Boys in Kansas City, Missouri, and
published a ground-breaking article, "Family Group Art
Therapy: Treatment of Choice for a Specific Case"
(Muller, 1968).

Robert Ault is now retired from the Menninger
Foundation. He initiated the undergraduate and graduate
art therapy programs at Emporia State University in
Emporia, Kansas, and has been a tireless presenter. He
is fond of talking about what he calls "the art therapy
movement." In recent years, he has helped bring to light
the artwork of Elizabeth Layton and pioneered the use of
art therapy with corporations and organizations. His
contributions to AATA have been numerous.[12] In 1985,
he was chosen Kansas State Educator of the Year. Felice

Cohen later became a president of AATA and continues to work as an art therapist and researcher in Houston.

Because of the efforts of Marge Howard, the American Association of Art Therapy was chartered in Oklahoma in 1969, which was also the site of the first Executive Board meeting (Figure 14). Dues were set at $15.00. A roster dated in 1969 showed 20 members in good standing (Figure 15). Robert Ault, with the help of a graphic artist, designed AATA's logo.

The first *Newsletter* of the American Art Therapy Association, edited by Don Jones, contained the following "President's Message" from Myra Levick:

> For the past 20 years artists have been involved in using their skills to aid in the diagnosis and treatment of psychiatric patients and in more recent years have not only begun to speak and write about their experiences, but have been recognized for their contributions.
>
> It is an established fact that an organization must be formed in order to attain professional recognition. And it is with great pleasure that we announce that the AATA was voted into being on June 27, 1969, in Louisville, Kentucky, by a representative group of art therapists from all over the country and Canada. The goals of this new group go far beyond merely formalizing that which has already been achieved. It is hoped that Art Therapy and its relation to mental health and education will be more clearly defined and further developed. (Levick, 1970b, p. 1)

The First Conference

One hundred people attended AATA's first conference, held at Airlie House in Warrenton, Virginia, September, 1970. Margaret Naumburg was unanimously designated as the first recipient of an Honorary Life Membership[13] by the new AATA Executive Board. According to Ault, this was an effort to say: "We honor you, we respect you, we want you to be a part of us, but you cannot have control of us. We want you to join us" (Ault, 1975).

Even though she had stalked out of the organizational meeting in Philadelphia, Naumburg's warm acceptance of the Honorary Life Membership implied an endorsement of the new organization (Figure 16). Levick said:

> The highlight of the meeting [at Airlie] was Miss Naumburg's memorable acceptance speech...it was especially meaningful to many of us who knew this was the first and only professional group Miss Naumburg openly supported. Her words were insightful, professional, and inspiring. I treasure personal letters from her (sent to me as President of AATA) in which she stated how pleased she was with the directions we were taking to establish a field she had been committed to for many, many years. (Levick, 1975)

9 Top Art Therapists Plan for Future Here

By PAT ATKINSON
Of the World Staff

Nine national art therapists are meeting in Tulsa to hammer out the furure of their profession.

They are the executive committee of the newly formed American Art Therapy Association gathered for the first time to exchange ideas and provide structure to the lossely-knit profession.

"In the past there have always been pockets of activities over the country in art therapy, but each art therapist was in a sense isolated," explained Robert Ault, AATA president-elect and director of adjunctive therapies at the Menniger Foundation in Topeka.

"RIGHT NOW, WITH THE new organization, we're trying to establish things like criteria of registeration, working out guidelines for professional criteria," he said.

The group now has 54 active members and a mailing list of about 250 who are involved in some way with the field.

Ault said the field is growing rapidly and predicted a future involvement with universities. He has been teaching a graduate level seminar at the University of Kansas for students in art education.

"I think the future will find training af art therapists as a specialized education." Ault said. Traditionally, art students have studied under established practicing therapists in clinical facilities.

The field is a blend of art and psychology. Most therapists have a background in art that has lead to supplimental studies in psychology. Art therapy is generally part of a team approach to treating the mentally ill or emotionally disturbed.

"There is a difference in the degree and goals between teachers of art and art therapists," Ault said.

"ART IS A WAY OF GETting to the (problem) material, often subconscious, that is difficult to express verbally. Art therapy is based on something we all go through as children, with the symbolism, expression and communication," he said.

The officers will be meeting at the Camelot Inn through Friday. The meeting is under the local direction of Marge Howard, art therapist at the Children's Medical Center and treasurer of AATA.

Figure 14

119

AMERICAN ART THERAPY ASSOCIATION

1969 ROSTER

MEMBERS IN GOOD STANDING

1. Gladys L. Agell

    23 Vanderbilt Avenue
    Manhasset, New York

2. Brother Arthur C.S.C.

    151 South 84th Street
    Milwaukee, Wisconsin   53214

3. Robert E. Ault

    200 Western
    Topeka, Kansas

4. Lenore C. Bendheim
    (Student)

    509 Fireside Drive
    Apartment 9
    Lawrence, Kansas

5. Mrs. Felice W. Cohen

    3607 South Braeswood Blvd.
    Houston, Texas

6. Michelle LeMay Flesher

    628 Round Oak Road
    Towson, Maryland

7. Margaret C. Howard

    Box 7352
    Children's Medical Center
    Tulsa, Oklahoma   74105

8. Sandra Kagin

    600 South 31st
    Parsons, Kansas

9. Elsie E. Muller

    9801 Lee Blvd.
    Leawood, Kansas

10. Irmgard Hess Neiman

    1224 West Elmdale
    Chicago, Illinois

11. Lyzbeth Lynn Oliver
    (Student)

    Centennial Hall
    William Woods Collgeg
    Fulton, Missouri   65251

12. Kathleen E. Pellock

    2500 Belmont
    Parsons, Kansas

13. Ben J. Ploger
    (Life time)

    3224 De Soto Street
    New Orleans, Louisiana

14. D. Thresa Roach

    1625 Grand
    Parsons, Kansas

15. Kathleen Van Sickle   2334 Bowker Avenue
Victoria, B. C., Canada

16. Bernard O. Stone   1745 King
Apartment D
Columbus, Ohio

17. Elinor Ulman   Bulletin Art Therapy
6010 Broad Branch Road N.W.
Washington, D.C. 20015

18. Anne A. Wallace   7621 West 98th
     (Student)   Overland Park, Kansas 66212

19. Mrs. Myra Levick   Hahnemann Medical College & Hospital
314 North Broad Street
Philadelphia, Pennsylvania

20. Bernard Levy, Ph.D.   6010 Broad Branch Road, N.W.
George Washington
Professor of Psychology
Washington, D.C. 20015

Figure 15 (cont.)   121

MARGARET NAUMBURG
CERTIFIED PSYCHOLOGIST
135 EAST 54TH STREET
NEW YORK, N. Y. 10022
—
MURRAY HILL 8-6763

Feb, 22, 70

Mrs. Myra Levick, M. Ed,
Director, Art Therapy Program
The Hahnemann Medical College &
Philadelphia, Pa.   Hospital,

Dear Myra,

I feel greatly honored at being chosen to receive the plaque from the AATA as the first Honorary member of this organization, which was voted upon at the Louisville Kentucky meeting in June 1969,

With warm appreciation for this honor to the entire membership of AATA I am, sincerely yours,

Margaret

From its inception, the American Art Therapy Association, has been an organization of vital individualists with strong opinions and loud voices. The arguments through the years have been substantive, vocal and, at times, difficult and divisive. Judith Rubin, a past President of the Association, has written: "The early meetings were so full of passion and discord that I wondered whether I really wanted to be a part of this noisy group" (Rubin, 1985, p. 30). Harriet Wadeson put it this way:

> I attended the preliminary meeting in Philadelphia and the first conference at Airlie House outside Washington in 1970. I recall disagreeing with Margaret Naumburg on both occasions.... From the outset, I could see that we are certainly a group of "characters." (Wadeson, 1985, p. 31)

Elinor Ulman's account of that first annual meeting in the *American Journal of Art Therapy* (Volume 10, No. 1, 1970) elicited a number of angry letters from board members such as Felice Cohen (1970a), Myra Levick (1970a), and Bob Ault (1970) who felt that she presented a distorted view of what transpired. Levick's letter was printed in the *Journal*:

I have read your [EU's] account of the first annual conference...and must say that I am appalled by your biased
subjectivity and gross distortions.

...

...I cannot begin to comprehend what your editor's
note, "The Association is 14 years ahead of its time"
means. I do know that for many years the possibility of
forming a national art therapy organization has been discussed to no avail. Now, thanks to many people too numerous to list here, who are dedicated, involved and energetic, this organization has finally come about.

I hope this organization will continue to welcome
constructive criticism and diversified viewpoints. However, your particular criticism of the organization and its
officers has been destructive in its attempt to delay
progress. (Levick, 1971a, pp. 74, 99)

There were, however, letters taking Ulman's side.
Wayne Ramirez, president of the Wisconsin Art Therapy
Association, wrote to agree with her reporting (Ramirez,
1971a, p. 74; 1971b, p. 130). Herschel Stroyman
(1971, pp. 130, 143–144) said he "found Miss Ulman's
impressions...free of sycophancy, to the point, and
unanswered."

Developing Professional Standards

After the stormy sessions surrounding the formation of AATA, one of its first major battles concerned the question of registration. Social workers, with no available licensing in many states, had long awarded a national certification of competency by examination, designated by the letters ACSW (Academy of Certified Social Workers). Many other organizations also certified practitioners. At Warrenton, AATA voted to begin awarding registration[14] to those art therapists who could prove they met certain standards. The service mark would be A.T.R. for "Art Therapist, Registered." As President, Myra Levick wrote in the *AATA Newsletter*:

> The American Art Therapy Association took a giant step forward at its very first meeting in Warrenton, Virginia. The decision to certify art therapists under the Grandfather's Clause, who have been working in psychiatric settings for five years, was passed and the first registry will be published this year.
>
> An organization is recognized by the professional standards it maintains and aspires to. The decision to establish certification lays the groundwork for the development of these professional standards. It need not follow that every person using art in either education or psychiatric milieu would want to be certified. It is, however, important that the organization identify itself with specific goals. (Levick, 1970b, p. 1)

But the requirement of having worked in a psychiatric setting was one of the sticking points with some members who saw it as a premature narrowing of the field. In a letter to the editor in the *Bulletin*, Arthur Robbins stated that the Pratt Institute art therapy staff "recognize[d] the problems inherent in drawing up a certification for a discipline that has not yet crystallized" (Robbins, 1971, p. 100). By the time of the publication of the 1970 *Newsletter*, 52 of the 61 art therapists who qualified had written and accepted. However, Edith Kramer, wrote to say she did not want certification.[15] In a letter published in the *Newsletter*, Kramer stated her objections:

> There seem to be several reasons why certification is being sought. Important before all is the hope of enhancing the art therapist's bargaining power on the labor market. However, it seems to me unlikely that certification of art therapists by other art therapists would carry much weight in any struggle for better pay or for respect and recognition on the job. Attempts at obtaining certification from the outside, on the other hand, would entail a great deal of preparatory work on our part in defining the profession. It seems to me that any ill-prepared moves in this direction would be likely to jeopardize our ultimate goal.
>
> I therefore see no other reason to rush to certification other than the desire to quickly establish standards of ex-

cellence amongst art therapists. Certification, however, seems to me to be apt to induce premature rigidity within a field that must remain flexible and open to experimentation if it is to grow and to prove its worth.

...As a member of the editorial board of the *American Journal of Art Therapy*, I have had the often painful duty to read manuscripts written by persons without academic titles as well as by others who had obtained the right to add all kinds of letters to their names, including "PhD" and "MD." This experience has taught me that the possession of degrees of any kind constitutes no guarantee whatever of the ability to think clearly or to write grammatically....

To summarize, I am of the opinion that in order to obtain the right to establish standards and to invent titles, art therapists must give themselves more time to discuss, experiment and learn. (Kramer, 1970)

In her argument, Kramer neglected to recognize the model of most professional groups, including doctors and lawyers which set up their own qualifying exams and enforce quality control. Felice Cohen, AATA's Secretary answered Kramer's letter by stating:

The rationale behind certification and registration was precisely to remove rigidity within the field. Up to this time, art therapy has been quite rigid. There have been so few who were included into what was a rather small group of art therapists. Those art therapists were mostly located in the East. There has been only one publication for art therapists, the *American Journal of Art Therapy*. Now, there is another publication, the *AATA Newsletter*...there is now diversification in the field...more people can be heard. Since the formation of AATA, we have qualified art therapists from practically every state in the country and Canada. This can be construed as flexibility. (Cohen, 1970b, p. 2)

Not only had there been a tremendous battle at the conference on the question of having professional standards for registration at all, but there were major differences in what kind of standards to have and how to proceed. The two groups collided with each other philosophically and with vehemence. Judith Rubin remembers:

[Kramer and Ulman] were worried that what they (and Naumburg) had conceptualized would be prematurely narrowed. There were no villians or heros, but everyone was very passionate and wanted to insure the survival of the profession to which they had given their life's blood. But they had different ideas of how to get there. Somewhat later, in Houston at a meeting of the American Society for Psychopathology of Expression, a group of us had lunch and Sandra Graves came up with a wonderful compromise[16] which made it possible for people pursuing alternative avenues in art therapy education and experience to be considered to meet standards for registration and the argument was resolved. (Rubin, 1994, personal communication)

What has held the organization together during its wars and its relatively short life has been the overriding commitment on the part of the pioneers to the development of art therapy as a therapeutic discipline. Like a vital, opinionated, competitive family, the members argued. But like a family, they often formed into a protective circle to fight the important battles necessary to carry the profession forward. Whatever else might be said about the American Art Therapy Association, it could never be called dull! And one of the major battles within AATA has been that of the definition of art therapy itself.

DEFINING ART THERAPY

Problems of defining[17] art therapy have intrigued and plagued the field since its inception and have continued to be a major concern of the American Art Therapy Association. With Naumburg and Kramer, the two major theorists, focusing on different definitions of the process, art therapists have often argued vehemently for one position or the other and have differed over whether to have a narrow or inclusive definition.[18] While this division has been perceived by many as a political one, initially, at least, it was an argument over where the cure was in art therapy treatment. Naumburg and Kramer took seemingly opposite positions. Naumburg's definition of art therapy as "a method of releasing the unconscious by means of spontaneous art expression" was countered by Kramer who described art as "a means of widening the range of human experiences by creating equivalents for such experiences. It is an area wherein experiences can be chosen, varied, and repeated at will"[19] (1958, p. 8).

Kramer contends: "The art therapist assists in an act of integration and synthesis which is performed by the ego" (Kramer, 1958, p. 21). Fink, Levick, and Goldman defined art therapy within a medical model as "that discipline which combines elements of psychotherapy with untapped sources of creativity and expression in the patient" (Fink, Levick, & Goldman, 1967, p. 2). Levick, from a decidedly Freudian perspective, further asserts that

> art therapy should be considered a prescribed substitution of creative activity to replace neurotic symptoms and to strengthen defenses successfully by the patient before illness becomes acute, and establish a prescribed relationship with the therapist. (Levick, 1967, p. 158)

Ulman discussed the question of definition and finally came down at a middle position:

My point of view is very strongly that art therapy does and should continue to mean a range of activities and at one end it begins to touch on art education...at the other end of the range it touches very closely on psychotherapy and psychotherapeutic uses of visual material. I feel hopeful that it can be established that this is a range of activities and not a hierarchy of activities. (1975a)

Moving more toward a Kramerian stance, Ulman goes on to say:

For art therapy to exist and grow as an independent discipline really depends on something within this range on the art side rather than the psychotherapy side...this new profession depends for its existence on the unique values that can be found in art and the art experience. (1975a)

Don Jones (1975) defined what he saw as three separate facets of art therapy—the analytical, functional, and avocational. He viewed analytical art therapy as "approaching the patient with our awareness and psychoanalytic understanding of the dynamics...free association by word, but getting into dream and preconscious imagery and bringing this up." In functional art therapy, "for example, you have a patient whose feelings are locked and bound, art therapy is a method of unlocking and expressing, and insight can be gained from the imaginal realm as well as from the cognitive and verbal level" (Jones, 1975). The third facet, avocational art therapy, provided "a therapeutic experience to learn how to paint and there are some patients who are treated using creative expression as a means of replacing narcissistic loss."

Another viewpoint was that of Mala Betensky, a psychologist and art therapist, who uses a phenomenological psychology framework. She postulates a type of art therapy in which the art experience provides an experiential source of self-awareness "to help the individual discover his authentic self" (Betensky, 1973, p. xi).

In *The Gestalt Art Experience*, Janie Rhyne placed Gestalt psychology within a humanistic theoretical framework to provide yet another definition. Rhyne concluded that:

> Gestalt art experience, then, is the complex personal you making art forms, being involved in the forms you are creating as events, observing what you do, and hopefully perceiving through your graphic productions not only yourself as you are now, but also alternate ways that are available to you for creating yourself as you would like to be. (Rhyne, 1973, p. 9)

Obviously, each of the previous views describes a "part of the elephant."[20] As separate entities, all are correct and all are incomplete. In an early pamphlet of the American Art Therapy Association the goal of art therapy was explained as "help for the individual child or adult to find a more compatible relationship between his inner and outer worlds" (Levick, 1983a, p. 3). In the late 1970s, the American Art Therapy Association moved toward a broader and more inclusive definition:

> Art therapy provides the opportunity for nonverbal expression and communication. Within the field there are two major approaches. The use of art as therapy implies that the creative process can be a means both of reconciling emotional conflicts and of fostering self-awareness and personal growth. When using art as a vehicle for psychotherapy, both the product and the associative references may be used in an effort to help the individual find a more compatible relationship between his inner and outer worlds.
>
> Art therapy like art education may teach technique and media skills. When art is used as therapy the instruction provides a vehicle for self-expression, communication and growth. Less product oriented, the art therapist is more concerned with the individual's inner experience. Process, form, content and/or associations become important for what each reflects about personality development, personality traits and the unconscious. (American Art Therapy Association pamphlet, 1977)

Finally, in 1985, a job description was written by Maxine Borowsky Junge, then AATA's first Chair of the Clinical Committee.[21]

THE DEVELOPMENT OF FORMAL EDUCATION FOR ART THERAPISTS

Early Education

The early art therapists found training in a variety of ways, often through their connections with psychiatrists or psychiatric clinics and often "on the job," inventing new strategies and techniques as they went along. Then they began to train others, as did Hanna Yaxa Kwiatkowska at the National Institute of Mental Health with her student Harriet Wadeson. Margaret Naumburg's art therapy traveling "road show," in which she presented her work in many geographical areas and to many professional groups, served to make her the voice of art therapy. Gary Barlow, formerly Director of Art Therapy at Wright State University in Dayton, Ohio, remembers his role as the excited young student who picked up Naumburg at the airport when she came to speak at Miami University in Oxford, Ohio in 1957 (G. Barlow, personal communication, 1985). Her talks inspired and sparked interest in many to seek some kind of formal education. Naumburg is said to have trained a number of art therapists, but the exact form of this training is unclear, until the instigation of what she termed "the first course introducing principles and methods of art therapy" in a university setting to graduate students at New York University in 1958 (Naumburg, 1966, p. 32).

Various Approaches

In its first years, the American Art Therapy Association undertook the important task of developing standards for national registration. Those who designed the standards wisely recognized that few formal opportunities for art therapy education existed. And indeed, there were few art therapists to help in that education; in many parts of the country, there were none. At the beginning, AATA designated a wide variety of educational approaches such as self-education, apprenticeships, inservice hospital training, and university programs to gain registration. However, when AATA began to make education specifically in art therapy a requirement for registration it, along with growing interest in art therapy nationwide, helped launch a tremendous growth of academic, clinical, and institute training programs in the 1970s.

Art therapy education was driven by a number of historical factors. It was a time of remarkable innovation and energy, born out of the alternative education philosophies of the late 1960s and the insistence on making education relevant to life and self-direction on the part of university students of the time. Further, the human potential movement of the 1960s had given rise to a generation interested in exploring the values of self-understanding through diverse new therapies.

Also influential in the rapid development of art therapy education was the movement to take the mentally ill out of the back wards and return them to their home communities where it was believed that they could be treated more humanely and effectively.[22] Under President John F. Kennedy, legislation was enacted to develop community mental health centers. The funnelling of immense amounts of money and expertise into the centers gave rise to an emphasis on innovation in treatment approaches. As a result, many enthusiastic people sought formal training as psychotherapists, psychiatric social workers, psychologists, and art therapists. But, arguments raged about the type of education necessary for the art therapy community. Edith Kramer, calling herself an "inveterate rebel of the old school," wrote in a letter to Felice Cohen (Kramer, 1971a) arguing against academic "mills":

> We must be equally concerned with the destiny of the intuitive artistic individual who can function exquisitely with people and with art materials but has no aptitude for book learning. To push such persons through the academic mill is destructive both to them and to academic standards that are lowered by the influx of inadequately educated students. Instead, our profession must find ways of training such people's natural aptitudes by *other means*. We must defend their right to work rather than crowd them out by making employment increasingly dependent on academic degrees only.
>
> In making these points, I do not mean to denigrate an academic course of training, such as developed by Hahnemann and other sites of learning. Nor do I mean to imply that such training need necessarily stifle original thinking. I do feel that it is essential that alternate possibilities of entering the profession should be developed to supplement the academic one.
>
> I can imagine that many readers will find my ideas too impractical. Art therapy, so they say, must come to terms with existing conditions, such as an increasing demand for academic degrees. The members' eagerness in seeking registration even now when the organization is comparatively powerless is a measure of their anxiety and desire for some form of organizational support and protection. In my opinion, it is essential that such support should not be paid for by subservience to a narrow set of artificial values that is becoming increasingly destructive to the life

of our society, and would divorce us from vital sources of creative energy. How to find a way of implementing a broader definition of art therapy and make it acceptable on the labor market is, I admit, a difficult question, but one that must be faced.

As for myself, I should become a registered member of the AATA only if I were assured that the profession admits, besides the student possessing the required degrees, also members of the black community and indeed of all groups existing beyond the pale of the white American middle class.

On the whole, I am distressed by the tendency in our profession to define the field of art therapy exclusively by academic standards. Such a development would exclude two kinds of people: on the one hand, the intellectually gifted, self-directed person who is able to acquire knowledge by intelligent reading and to perceive patterns and formulate concepts from the raw material of experience but who cannot tolerate the treadmill of conventional academic procedures and whose creative capacities are stifled by the classroom atmosphere; on the other hand, the intuitive person, gifted in working with people and with art materials who has no talent or interest in book learning or whose education has been so neglected that book learning is bound to remain alien to him.

I myself belong to the first category. Having had an excellent basic education in a Viennese *Realgymnasium*, I was, upon graduation at age eighteen, well equipped to acquire knowledge independently as I become interested in a subject. Naturally, this pertains to the humanities only, for evidently I could not have become competent in professions such as medicine or chemistry without submitting to the necessary technical training in approved institutes of learning. Essential in my development as an art therapist was my training as an artist (also arrived at beyond the pale of Academia) and my continued devotion to my artistic pursuits, my personal psychoanalysis, and years of experience as an art therapist and teacher in situations that brought me in contact with professionals knowledgeable in related disciplines whose observations and advice I would absorb and apply in manners suitable to my chosen field. I know that I should never have entered the field of art therapy had I been required to follow a conventional course of academic training. I feel that it is essential that the door should remain open to others who, like myself, are too eccentric, too passionately devoted to their own purposes, too disillusioned with the academic establishment, or for other reasons unwilling to acquire the well informed rebellious mind lacking degrees and the academically inadequate working person who compensates for it by unusual capacities in practical work.

Thank you for permitting an inveterate rebel of the old school expression in your publication.

> Very sincerely yours,
> Edith Kramer
> (February 25, 1971)

Myra Levick, then AATA President, wrote to Kramer on November 9, 1971:

Every organization must begin somewhere. In the history of all organizations a group of professionals come together, set up preliminary standards, and certify their colleagues. As this body grows, they become a power to seek recognition and accreditation from those organizations that have this right. You are quite right—a great deal of preparatory work is indeed necessary in order to define the profession and seek outside certification. Some of this work has already been done here at Hahnemann and hopefully, more is being done by other people connected with our organization. For example, we have prepared a comprehensive detailed application to the American Medical Association for recognition of the training program here. Our constitution and by-laws make it clear that art therapy in a mental institution or a school for emotionally disturbed children is only one area in which members of the American Art Therapy Association can achieve some of the goals of the professional. Flexibility of the field is protected by our constitution. I am well aware of your particular experience, and would like to suggest that you design an outline for a course to include some of your ideas. I might add that the course here at Hahnemann is by no means limited to applicants from any single socioeconomic class. We are accredited for all education loans and yet have been unable to attract any poor people or black people. We have been fortunate enough to have three male students in the last 3 years. I agree with you, there is much to be said against the acquiring of degrees. Nevertheless, this is the system, and until we can come up with a better one, we have no choice but to meet those presently in existence in the "better universities" in the country.

Art therapists cannot experiment and learn unless there are environments for them to learn in. Therefore, I repeat my above statement—we must start somewhere, and the fact that there are now two master's degree programs established, I think, is a good beginning. I look forward to hearing from you and having your ideas in writing so that through the organization and interested institutions we may begin to explore the possibilities of developing them.

Sincerely yours,
(Mrs.) Myra Levick,
President

By 1992, there were 32 Master's degree programs to educate art therapists across the country and numerous courses both undergraduate and graduate. In addition, there was clinical training in hospital settings and freestanding institutes were on the rise. However, the stringencies of the economic crisis nationwide was also beginning to take its toll as universities cut back, and two approved programs of long standing, Wright State and State University of New York at Buffalo, closed. Perhaps this is a forewarning of an important and disturbing future ahead for art therapy education.

By the early 1970s, the American Art Therapy Association had developed guidelines for the education of art therapists which included both didactic courses and practicum experience.

After a number of Master's degree programs evolved nationwide, it was generally considered that the Master's degree was the desired entry level into the profession. However, the American Art Therapy Association did not make this a requirement until 1993. There is controversy over which graduate program was first. The program instituted at the University of Louisville in 1957 by Dr. Roger White had at least two graduates in 1959 before it fell into inactivity for 10 years. Located in both the Psychology Department and the Department of Art, the program was revived in June, 1969. In 1973, this program became independent within the university as the Institute for Expressive Therapies. This move toward inter-disciplinary expressive therapy studies would provide another point of continuing debate for the field as many would see it as a dilution of what had not yet proved itself as a separate discipline.

Due to Paul Fink's and Morris Goldman's enthusiasm for art therapy, Hahnemann Medical College (later University) and Hospital in Philadelphia hired Myra Levick as Director of Adjunctive Therapies and coordinator of a graduate-level program which began in September, 1967. This was three months before the organizational meeting held by Hahnemann which led to the formation of the American Art Therapy Association.

Levick calls this "the first training program anywhere to offer graduate-level training leading to a Master's degree in art therapy" (Levick, 1986, p. 187). For two years, Edith Kramer was one of the instructors. Soon after, a program was introduced at the George Washington University in Washington DC, administered by Dr. Bernard Levy with Elinor Ulman.[23] Teaching at George Washington along with Ulman and Levy were Hanna Yaxa Kwiatkowska and Edith Kramer, who commuted from New York City.

The next training program was initiated in 1970 by Dr. Josef E. Garai at the Pratt Institute, a free-standing art school in New York. Garai attended the second annual conference of the American Art Therapy Association in Milwaukee, Wisconsin, where he presented a paper called "The Humanistic Approach to Art Therapy and Creativity Development." Garai based his theoretical approach on a humanistic psychology framework and described his work as "client centered and client oriented" (1985, p. 27). He describes the response to his paper:

> The younger members of the Association were showing by their enthusiastic applause how much they favored this new and unconventional approach. But in the ensuing discussion, I saw myself confronted by attacks orchestrated by the "Old Guard" who regarded this theory as

heresy and insisted on the traditional psychoanalytic approach[24].... Soon afterwards I was denounced as a "troublemaker, rebel and crazy person." (1985, p. 27)

Born in Germany, Garai earned his doctorate in social psychology and personality from New York University in 1959. At Pratt, Garai instituted the first humanistically oriented art therapy program under a Master of Professional Studies degree program. He founded the art therapy program at Pratt in 1970 and then the dance/movement therapy programs in 1978.

After a few years it became the biggest training program in the country and attracted students from most of the states of the USA and from all over the world...during my tenure [1970–1980] Pratt Institute graduated 450 students with master's degrees in art therapy. (Garai, 1985, p. 28)

Garai became Professor Emeritus in 1980. He defined humanistic art therapy thusly:

The humanistic approach to art therapy and creativity development is based on three fundamental assumptions. The first assumption states that people rather than being called mentally ill are likely to encounter specific problems in coping with life as a result of intrapsychic and environmentally caused conflicts. Treatment must be directed toward the reinforcement of the will to live and the development of the ability to find meaning and identity in as fully creative a life style as possible. The second assumption implies that the inability to cope successfully with the vicissitudes of life or to find satisfactory avenues toward self-actualization, meaning, and identity is a common phenomenon affecting most people to a greater or lesser degree at different stages of their lives. At any rate, it is not a sign of mental illness but rather a process inherent in the struggle to establish stability and continuity in an ever more rapidly changing and confusing macrocosmic and microcosmic environment. Instead of waiting to "cure" people whose ability to cope has been greatly decreased, creative-expressive approaches inherent in the mislabeled field of "art therapy" can and must be applied in working with all people. Such preventive application can provide the types of life experience which enhance curiosity, excitement, self-expression, and genuine intimacy. Such mass applications of principles of creativity development necessitate the replacement of the term "art therapy" by some more adequate concept emphasizing positive aspects rather than illness. Some of the suggested terms describing this type of creativity development are "self-expression through art," "creative artistic self-actualization," or "creative-expressive life-styling." (Garai, 1971, pp. 7–8)

The fifth program and the first on the West Coast was developed by Helen Landgarten at Immaculate Heart College in Los Angeles in 1973. At that time, Immaculate Heart was nationally known as a center of creativity in education and its art department was particularly renowned.[25] Landgarten's program, however, was not connected administratively to the college's art department, but was the first separate Department of Art Therapy in the country. From her training as a primary therapist in an outpatient community mental health center, Landgarten designed a curriculum intended to train art psychotherapists with the emphasis on the psychotherapy part as Naumburg had stressed. She called her program "Clinical Art Therapy" and focused on the visual arts. During their two-year education the Immaculate Heart students undertook more than 800 hours of supervised practicum and graduated able to function as primary therapists who, depending on the needs of the institution, could carry full case responsibility. When Immaculate Heart College closed in 1980, the Department moved to Loyola Marymount University, also in Los Angeles where it is today.

Also deserving of mention because of its unique focus is the art therapy program at Wright State University in Dayton, Ohio. Started by Gary Barlow in 1978 (and unfortunately closed in 1993), the program specialized in education for the treatment of clients with physical disabilities and trained many art therapists with physical disabilities.

One of the first hospital-based clinical training programs was initiated in the 1960s by Bernard Stone. Don Jones remembers meeting Stone at Menninger's:

> A young man came as a fine painter to ask about becoming an art therapist. I'm afraid I discouraged him but he was persistent and when I came to Ohio [to Harding Hospital in 1967] he was here. Bernard Stone had trained with a Dr. Pedro Corrons and they had established in the state hospital system a very sophisticated art psychotherapy training program. (Jones, 1975)

Pedro Corrons was a psychiatrist and a painter who had written the book *Colors of the Mind* (1973)[26] and established the first in-service clinical training program for art psychotherapy at Columbus State Hospital. Stone worked with Corrons at Columbus State and then moved on to the Good Samaritan Medical Center in Zanesville, Ohio.

By the mid-1970s, the American Art Therapy Association had established the Education and Training Board which was mandated to determine if programs met the educational guidelines set forth by the Association. By granting "Approved" status to certain programs the Association, while recognizing diverse philosophies and approaches, aimed to insure a high level of education for art therapists and protection for their clients.

In 1975 another important event in the evolution of art therapy education occurred; the first conference for art therapy educators was held in Washington, DC, hosted by the George Washington University. About 20 people attended.[27] This conference addressing issues important to the education of art therapists continues to be held approximately biennially. It has attracted educators from across the country and Europe and is now known as the International Convocation of Art Therapy Educators.

The education list published by the American Art Therapy Association in 1990 included 21 Approved programs (one clinical and one institute training program), 24 universities and colleges offering art therapy programs and courses, two graduate-level certificate programs, five clinical programs, five institute programs and 28 universities and colleges offering undergraduate art therapy degree programs offering art therapy prerequisites.[28]

Notes:

[1] AATA's exclusive right to use this service mark was challenged by another association but was upheld in

federal court in 1990 (see the President's Letter in the *AATA Newsletter*, 1991, Vol. XXIV, No. 1, p. 1).

[2] The community mental health centers were established by the Community Mental Health Act (Public Law 88-164) passed in 1963.

[3] Art therapy (along with dance therapy and music therapy) was mentioned in the regulations for Public Law 94–142 (the Education for All Handicapped Act).

[4] Née Graves.

[5] Those art therapists included Naumburg, Jane Gilbert, Lynn Berger, Carolyn Refsnes Kniazzeh, Hanna Yaxa Kwiatkowska, Miryam Dergalis, and Myra Levick.

[6] Boston was the site of the "first all-day conference" on art therapy, January 15, 1966, organized by Carolyn Refsnes and Vernon Patch, MD. Three hundred people attended (*Bulletin of Art Therapy, 5,* 116–121).

[7] Née Refsnes.

[8] Levick served in that capacity from 1969 to 1971.

9 Much of the following information has been collected from the archives of the American Art Therapy Association housed at the Menninger Foundation, Topeka, Kansas. The original documents in the figures are also from the Archives.

10 To further her argument, Ulman published an article by Stern and Honoré (1969) on the problems and questions entailed in the formation of an association entitled "The Problem of National Organization: Make Haste Slowly."

11 See the Appendix for that document.

12 In addition to being AATA's second President (1971–1973) Ault was the Chair of the Education and Training Board.

13 Later recipients of the Honorary Life Membership Award honoring significant contributions to the field were Edith Kramer, Myra Levick, Elinor Ulman, Bernard Levy, Helen Landgarten, Elsie Muller, Hanna Yaxa Kwiatkowska, Rawley Silver, Judith Rubin, Janie Rhyne, Gladys Agell, Robert Ault, Don Jones, Felice Cohen, Frances Anderson, Cay Drachnik, Harriet Wadeson, and Gwen Gibson.

[14] Registration is one of the lower levels of professional credentialing since it is based on education and experience but not on demonstrated competencies. A more stringent level of credentialing is based on a national examination. In all professional organizations, the requirements for credentialing are gradually tightened as the discipline develops.

[15] Others who were offered registration under a grandparenting arrangement but originally refused were Janie Rhyne and Arthur Robbins.

[16] Graves' suggestion was to award applicants for registration Professional Quality Credits (PQCs) based on their education and training, with different experiences being given a different number of points. One had to amass a total of 12 PQCs in order to be granted registration.

[17] For other discussions on the definition of art therapy see Ault, 1977; McNiff, 1979; Shoemaker, 1977; Kramer & Ulman, 1976; and Ulman, 1992 [originally published in 1961; see Ulman (1961b)].

[18] One debate centered on whether one should be a generalist who uses several art forms or a specialist

who uses only the visual arts (Agell & McNiff, 1982).

19 Elinor Ulman uses this quotation in her paper on definition but she adds the following sentence to Kramer's statement: "In the creative act, conflict is re-experienced, resolved and integrated." This addition has been retained in reprints of Ulman's article.

20 Rubin (1987c) uses this analogy in her book on various theoretical approaches to art therapy.

21 See Appendix.

22 This emphasis on returning patients to the community is now seen by many as resulting in the increasing numbers of homeless in American cities. The community services necessary for such a program were often inadequate or unavailable.

23 This program developed out of the art therapy courses Elinor Ulman was giving at the Washington School of Psychiatry. In 1970, the University started a Master's in Special Studies program. In 1971, the program became a full-fledged Master of Arts in Art Therapy.

24 Gantt (1991, personal communication) stated: "I think that Garai was trying to set himself apart from those he thought were interpreting art in a mechanistic unvarying fashion."

25 This was because of the work of Sister Mary Corita, a young nun who later became known as Corita Kent. Her clear, vibrant, and playful serigraphed images combining abstract form and color with words and quotations made an important impact on the art world and helped to expand graphic and advertising design.

26 We have been unable to find more detailed publication information on this book. It was mentioned in the September 1973 issue of *Voice*, the AATA newsletter (Vol. III, No. 3, pp. 6–7), but no publisher was listed.

27 This writer (MBJ) attended. My memories are of the thrill of meeting many of the art therapists whom I had long admired through their writings and watching them argue their points of view with such vehemence and, at times, venom that I was astounded and distressed.

28 The current Education List may be obtained through the AATA office.

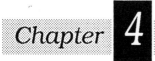

The Art Therapy Literature

With the rapidly increasing interest in art therapy and the burgeoning of training programs, it was inevitable that there has been a proliferation of art therapy literature since the early 1970s. This chapter surveys the literature that became the foundation for the field and includes the major books published up to 1990.

Journals & Annotated Bibliographies

[By 1960, Margaret Naumburg and Edith Kramer had formulated their theoretical bases for art therapy.] With her creation of the first journal in 1961, Elinor Ulman provided an avenue for communication and the exchange of ideas and techniques. In 1973, Ernest Harms,[1] a psychiatrist, established a second journal[2] named *Art*

Psychotherapy which included dance/movement, poetry, music, and drama as well as the visual arts in therapy. This journal was edited by Harms until his death in 1974 when Paul Jay Fink and Edith Wallace, both psychiatrists, became editors. In 1980, the name of the journal was changed to *The Arts in Psychotherapy*. Both Myra Levick and David Read Johnson, a psychologist and drama therapist, have served as Editor-in-Chief. The current editor is Robert Landy, a drama therapist.

In 1983, the *American Journal of Art Therapy* ended its affiliation[3] with the American Art Therapy Association and negotiated an arrangement to be published by Norwich University in Vermont. Also in 1983, AATA began its own journal, *Art Therapy*, under interim editors Linda Gantt and Mildred Lachman-Chapin. Gary Barlow served as editor from 1983 to 1991, succeeded by Cathy Malchiodi.

Linda Gantt and Marilyn Schmal compiled an annotated bibliography of art therapy literature covering the years 1940 to 1973 (Gantt & Schmal, 1974).[4] This booklet and a subsequent one, *Art Therapy in Mental Health*, compiled by Rosanna Moore (1981), were published by the National Institute of Mental Health. The needs of students along with the increasing sophistication of pioneer art therapists and their wish to share their work with others created a profusion of art therapy literature from a variety of viewpoints. Much of this was in the form of descriptive case studies which dramatically and visually portrayed the various uses and techniques and the value of art therapy. Many early training programs relied heavily on literature from psychology and psychoanalysis because, for the most part, that was all that existed. Thus, it was essential to the evolving discipline that new generations of art therapists have their elders and role models available to them through their writings. During this period, art therapists were often invited to contribute material to psychological and psychotherapeutic books and journals. Certainly, not all the art therapy literature can be surveyed here, but what follows represents a cross-section of the important early works with a foray into the second-generation authors.[5]

This section is divided into two parts: psychoanalytic and psychodynamic perspectives, and alternative perspectives. A chronology in the Appendix lists the writers and their first publications.

Psychoanalytic & Psychodynamic Perspectives: The First Generation

Margaret Naumburg:
Dynamically Oriented Art Therapy

Margaret Naumburg[6] had a broad and wide-ranging interest in a number of fields which bordered art therapy.[7] Indicative of the depth of her scholarship are the summaries of relevant American and European literature she provided in her major books (1950, 1953, 1966) which place art therapy within a theoretical as well as historical perspective. She drew freely from a range of sources and ideas and advocated that her trainees do the same. She contended that teachers and therapists could deal with unconscious material only "when they have acquired a thorough background in those concepts relating to the unconscious, which have been developed by Freud, Jung, Sullivan, Fromm, Erikson, and others" (Naumburg, 1966, p. 33).

In addition to incorporating these psychological concepts into her method of working she had a comprehensive view of how art functioned in human history. Naumburg was convinced that "image-making was a vital form of communication in the life of early man" (p.

37) and that by understanding art from both an archaeological and an anthropological perspective art therapists could better understand their patients' art:

> Earlier cultures, which produced anonymous carvings of strange gods and mythical creatures, did so as a gesture of religious dedication, which is not to be confused with "art" in our modern sense. Only when we are able to relinquish temporarily our specialized focus on "art" can we relate ourselves to so different a view of life as is found in certain ancient and primitive cultures. (p. 37)

According to Naumburg, "dynamically oriented" art therapy relies on understanding how unconscious content is communicated through symbolic means. The art provides a concrete object to which the patient is asked to freely associate. While she took the technique of free association from psychoanalysis, Naumburg did not agree with the Freudians' stress on putting subjective experiences into words. In contrasting the two approaches Naumburg stated that "In art therapy the patient's unconscious imaged experience is transposed directly into an actual pictured image" whereas in psychoanalysis "such inner visual experiences must be retranslated from an imaged into a verbal communication" (p. 2). Unfortunately, this retranslation usually has a negative effect on the symbol.

When an interior experience of imaged symbols is thus consistently reduced to words, it has been deprived of certain aspects of its dynamism. For a pictured symbol... may have meanings that cannot be reduced to the spoken or written word. (Naumburg, 1950, p. 15)

It was a Freudian contention that symbolized material was always regressive in nature. But Naumburg endorsed Rollo May's idea that there could be a progressive aspect to symbols as well. May asserted that they "bring out new meaning, new forms, disclose reality, which was literally not present before" (May quoted by Naumburg, 1966, p. 21) and that this "progressive aspect...is almost completely omitted in the traditional Freudian psychoanalytic approach" (p. 21). Naumburg agreed that a symbol "reaches into dimensions beyond the intellectualized grasp of speech" (Naumburg, 1950, p. 16). Visual symbolism is "a natural, positive and normal form of nonverbal, imaged expression shared by both primeval and modern man" (Naumburg, 1966, p. 29). She asserted that both education and psychotherapy would be improved if teachers and therapists paid more attention to "the vital significance of imagery" (p. 29).

To illustrate that the reliance of the Freudians on the unvarying meaning of so-called universal symbols was too narrow, Naumburg cited the work of Ainslie Meares who distinguished a "fundamental difference" between universal and personal symbols (Naumburg, 1966, p. 28). Naumburg concurred with Meares that the meaning of some symbols could only be understood by listening to the patient's own interpretations, not by applying an inflexible theory.

Therefore, when it came to espousing a specific theory for interpreting artwork, Naumburg chose neither Jung nor Freud but instead suggested this third option of making the patient the interpreter.

> Regardless of the fact that Freud rejected and Jung accepted the use of symbolic expression in psychotherapy, dynamically oriented art therapy cannot be tied to any one specific scientific interpretation of the significance of spontaneous art or dream productions. Dynamically oriented art therapy leaves a patient free to direct his associations to the images he creates in any direction he chooses. It therefore frees the patient from overdependence on the art therapist and also speeds up the therapeutic procedure. (p. 22)

In her book *Schizophrenic Art: Its Meaning in Psychotherapy* (1950) Naumburg wrote a lengthy comparison of two case studies in which the patient's art was included, one by a therapist who used a Freudian approach and another by one who used a Jungian approach. She granted that "It is not improbable that a Freudian or Jungian patient tends to produce symbols in the style and form most acceptable to his therapist." But she continued:

> We have a right to question why, if the unconscious is truly universal, should such symbolic groupings of material seem inevitably to substantiate either a Freudian or Jungian analysis? Is it not possible that such interpretations of symbolism as are identified with each school of psychotherapy may contain richer and more extensive meanings than their special interpretations have so far suggested? And is it not possible to discover with the greater assistance of the patient what his own symbolic productions really mean to him, with less interpretation by the psychotherapist? (Naumburg, 1950, p. 21)

Such self-interpretation promotes the patient's cathexis to the art and paves the way to growth and autonomy.

This emphasis on the patient's capacity for interpreting his/her own work was more than an issue of declaring independence from a specific psychological theory; it provided a basis for justifying art therapy as a specific type of treatment: "For it is on the basis of each patient's response to his own symbolic creations that the importance of using spontaneous art projections as a primary mode of therapy can be established" (p. 34).

In Naumburg's method, the therapist is seen as a facilitator in an interpersonal relationship whose primary role is to encourage the patient to discover for him/herself the meaning of the art. Empathy, the encouragement of free association, and basic instruction of simple art techniques are the tools of the therapist.

> Practice in the use of the art media must be carefully explained to patients inexperienced in painting or drawing, so as to help them release their unconscious imaged projections. After a preliminary explanation to patients as to the several ways in which pastels can be employed to express changing moods and phantasies, they are given a practical demonstration of how to apply what is known as the "scribble" technique. (Naumburg, 1966, p. 15)

By stressing that the art is best understood as "symbolic speech" rather than looking at it as an aesthetic object, the art therapist creates a more relaxed atmosphere which promotes greater expression of conflicts and anxieties. "When the therapist convinces the patient that he accepts whatever the patient may express, the patient often begins to project in images what he dares not put into words" (p. 2).

Naumburg thought that art therapy always took place within the transference relationship[8] and that evidence of the transference feelings could be seen in both the visual and verbal communication. But the patient developed a cathexis to the art as well as the therapist. This "narcissistic cathexis" to the artwork eventually paved the patient's path to autonomy. The transference within art therapy was different from that which was fostered in psychoanalysis precisely because the patient was encouraged to make his/her own interpretations rather than to rely on those of the therapist.

> But the transference relation in art therapy is considerably modified by the introduction of spontaneous images, for with the projection of images the patient, by means of free association, begins to understand more clearly the original objectification of his conflicts, which may have begun in his earliest family relationships. (p. 8)

It was the release of those unconscious conflicts that was a fundamental goal of the therapy (p. 3).

The actual frequency of the art-making was determined by each person's circumstances: "How each patient may choose to employ spontaneous art expression depends on each patient's individual needs whether he uses it constantly or intermittently, or only during critical phases of therapy" (p. 17).

Naumburg thought that art therapy could be used with "a wide range of neurotic and psychotic adult patients, as well as emotionally disturbed adolescents and children" (p. 6). But she felt that working with a professional artist "involves a special type of difficulty" because of the unconscious resistance of the patient:

> At first he tends to draw entirely conscious designs which are technically knowledgeable but without significance as a release of unconscious conflicts. When, however, such an artist succeeds in creating his first truly spontaneous image, he is usually eager to develop it into an artistically finished picture. He must then be made to understand that, in order to deal with his unconscious motivation, such imagery must be regarded as a form of symbolic speech to which he must learn to make free association. The artist is told that when his therapy has been completed he will be free to use his spontaneous pictures in any way he chooses. (p. 4)

Naumburg cites several advantages of art therapy including: producing a visual image which defies defenses more easily and enables unconscious material to surface more quickly; speeding up therapy through the making of verbal associations to the image; and promoting the patient's verbal expressiveness (pp. 4–10).

Edith Kramer:
The Healing Power of Art

Edith Kramer[9] was the second major theorist in the formative years of art therapy. She established a counterpoint to Naumburg's art therapy theory through her focus on the creative process itself. In describing "a fundamental cleavage" in art therapy Kramer stated her position thusly:

> Some art therapists practice it as a specialized form of psychotherapy, but here we are concerned mainly with art therapy that depends on *art* as its chief therapeutic agent. Art therapy is seen as distinct from psychotherapy. Its healing potentialities depend on the psychological processes that are activated in creative work. (Kramer, 1971b, p. 25, emphasis in the original)

Kramer developed her therapeutic methods working with disturbed boys at the Wiltwyck School for Boys in the 1950s. She is the author of many articles (1961, 1962, 1963, 1964, 1965, 1966, 1967, 1968, 1972, 1986, 1992b; Kramer & Scher, 1983; Kramer & Ulman, 1976; Kramer & Ulman, 1977) and three books, *Art Therapy in a Children's Community* (1958), *Art as Therapy with Children* (1971b), and *Childhood and Art Therapy* (1979). She has taught art therapy courses and workshops at the New School for Social Research and

Turtle Bay Music School and is presently teaching graduate art therapy courses at New York University and occasionally at the George Washington University.

Kramer's approach is based on Freudian psychoanalytic theory, but instead of concentrating on the resolution of intrapsychic conflict as Naumburg did, she focuses on strengthening the ego by promoting the defense mechanism of sublimation:

> Sublimation...is a process in which an instinctual aim is denied direct gratification. The original aim is replaced by a new, socially acceptable aim through a process which includes repression and reaction formation. The instinctual energy which is not discharged becomes, at least in part, available to the ego, is used in the development of skills and accomplishments which give the individual greater mastery over his environment and improve his capacity for positive object relationship so that he becomes a more valuable member of society. The gratification from the accomplishment replaces the instinctual gratification....
>
> With maturity and the establishment of the superego, sublimation becomes the ego's most economical method of reconciling the demands of the superego with instinctual demands. As the ego succeeds in forming a superstructure through which forbidden sexual and aggressive drives can find some measure of gratification through socially productive acts, gratification becomes possible with the approval of the superego. The ego succeeds in its function as an integrating force and is rewarded by a feeling of peace and achievement. (Kramer, 1958, pp. 13-14)

Having a thorough understanding of Freudian theory, Kramer is aware of "psychic process" and the "unconscious" but in her therapy does not emphasize these. Instead, her goal in art therapy is to support and foster growth of the ego and to help the child develop a sense of identity through creative involvement in art making.

To promote "systematic thinking" about the ways in which children can use art materials, Kramer describes what she sees as five different types of activity:

1. Precursory activities: scribbling, smearing; exploration of physical properties of the material that does not lead to creation of symbolic configurations but is experienced as positive and egosyntonic.
2. Chaotic discharge: spilling, splashing, pounding; destructive behavior leading to loss of control.
3. Art in the service of defense: stereotyped repetition; copying, tracing, banal conventional production.
4. Pictographs: pictorial communications which replace or supplement words....
5. Formed expression, or art in the full sense of the word; the production of symbolic configurations that successfully serve both self-expression and communication. (Kramer, 1971b, p. 54)

This final type of activity is the therapist's ultimate goal although Kramer admits that it is not always attainable (p. 66).

Since Kramer stresses the power of the creative process, interpretation of unconscious processes is not employed as a therapeutic tool. Rather, she attempts to understand the child's psychological functioning and offers interventions according to the clues she gets from behavior. Kramer is at the same time an art therapist and an art teacher. She creates an atmosphere where art can flourish, so that therapy becomes more conducive to art making.

> The basic aim of the art therapist is to make available to disturbed persons the pleasures and satisfactions which creative work can give and by his insight and therapeutic skill to make such experiences meaningful and valuable to the total personality. (Kramer, 1958, pp. 5-6)

Kramer argues that an art therapist has to be a "competent artist with specialized skills in the field of psychotherapy and education" (p. 7). Some of those specialized skills include "technical skill, pictorial imagination, ingenuity, and capacity to improvise" (Kramer, 1986, p. 71) and are used when offering a "Third Hand" to assist in the art making.

According to Kramer, the therapeutic relationship in art therapy is less intimate than in psychotherapy. The transference centers around the student's work and thus is not central to the therapeutic relationship. Nevertheless, Kramer is well aware that both transference and countertransference feelings occur in the art therapy sessions.

> Even though the development of transference in the full sense does not occur in art therapy, the therapist must understand the phenomenon. ... the universal inclination to respond to the present in terms of the past is particularly powerful among disturbed persons. Whatever relationships the art therapist establishes will therefore inevitably be colored by the children's transference, and it is likely, too, that his own responses will occasionally be contaminated by his counter-transference. (Kramer, 1971b, p. 39)

Kramer places great emphasis on the artistic quality of the art product. "After all," she said, "I am an artist and art teacher. I am not a psychologist" (personal communication, 1990). In a number of articles (1961, 1962, 1963, 1966, 1967, 1986) she has discussed the problems of quality in artwork and suggested ways for art therapists to deal with these problems.

Elinor Ulman:
The Voice of Art Therapy

Elinor Ulman[10] had a background in landscape architecture, drawing, and painting, and was a Phi Beta Kappa graduate of Wellesley College (Williams, 1992, p. 66). For 10 years she worked at the District of Columbia General Hospital and formed a great friendship with Bernard I. Levy, the chief psychologist. Together, they started the art therapy program at the George Washington University in 1971. From 1957 to 1973 she taught art therapy courses at the Washington School of Psychiatry. In 1961, Ulman created the *Bulletin of Art Therapy*, the only art therapy journal at the time. The *Bulletin* changed its name to the *American Journal of Art Therapy* in 1970.

Ulman's theoretical foundation is psychoanalytic:

> I had entered analysis shortly before my first foray into art therapy. The three analysts I eventually saw, though to varying degrees unorthodox, gave their primary allegiance to Freud. Certainly, my hours on the couch were not devoted to the discussion of rival psychological theories or rival philosophies of life, but it seems likely that my analysts' attitudes exerted influence in my eventual adoption of a generally Freudian outlook. (Ulman, 1987, p. 285)

Like Kramer, Ulman focused her work on the concept of sublimation. Speaking of the instinctual drives which sublimation tames Ulman says:

> The steam of instinctual energy is indeed dissipated in neurotic symptoms; in sublimation this same energy drives an engine that does useful work.... The marvel is that out of inevitable inner conflict, out of the same primeval forces so easily turned to violence and destruction, springs man's capacity for civilized living and the greatest cultural achievement. (Ulman, 1975b, p. 9)

While Ulman recognized the phenomenon of transference she did not encourage its deliberate cultivation.

> Art therapists who are really expert in their own province can offer something that psychoanalysts and other kinds of specialists in the "talking cures" cannot: the opportunity to experience the kind of functioning that is possible only in the process of making art works and to gain insights that may be obtained through this kind of experience and in no other way. With this end in view, the art therapist must indeed understand transference and know how to deal with it. His aim will be to behave in such a way that transference interferes as little as possible with the making of art that contains and expresses basic conflicts. (Kramer & Ulman, 1976, p. 2)

She (and Kramer as well) stressed that the art therapist should promote a *therapeutic alliance* instead.

Ulman undertook the task of defining art therapy in a paper first published in 1961 (Ulman, 1961b): "I believe the realm of art therapy should be so charted as to accommodate endeavors where neither the term art not the term therapy is stretched so far as to have no real meaning" (Ulman, 1975b, p. 12). In describing art, she said:

> Its motive power comes from within the personality; it is a way of bringing order out of chaos—chaotic feelings and impulses within, the bewildering mass of impressions from without. It is a means to discover both the self and the world, and to establish a relation between the two. In the complete creative process, inner and outer realities are fused into a new entity. (p. 13)

According to Ulman, the art therapist's role is a broad one: "By making art activity available to those who can use it and works of art available to the entire institutional population (staff as well as patients), the therapist whose medium is art makes a far-reaching contribution" (Ulman, 1975c, p. 18).

It was during her time at D.C. General Hospital that she played a role in helping the psychologist to diagnose patients by providing additional nonverbal information through artwork. Ulman developed an assessment procedure "for collecting data in a single session to illuminate not only pathology but the resources of the whole personality" (p. 19). This assessment is now called the Ulman Personality Assessment Procedure (UPAP).[11] She contended that the art therapist could discover "hidden capacities in some of our patients that neither clinical observation nor projective testing had revealed" (Ulman, 1975d, p. 386). Her conclusions not only provided diagnostic information but often served to pinpoint the strong areas of a patient's personality which opened avenues to successful therapy.

The patient was asked to complete a series of four pictures. First, the patient was asked to use the art materials to make a picture. Then Ulman would suggest that the patient draw imaginary lines in the air using the whole body. This served to relax the patient and to break down inhibitions. This procedure was intended to facilitate the next task. The patient was asked to make rhythmic lines with eyes closed or averted from the paper. The patient was then asked to develop an image from the scribble lines. (Doing the exercises and developing an image from the scribble was used frequently by Florence Cane.) The last task was to choose between developing another drawing from a scribble or doing a drawing "starting...on a blank sheet of paper" (p. 364).

According to Ulman:

> The first drawing in each series tends to demonstrate a person's habitual modes of response. The exercise and scribble technique make for a lowering of defenses and the emergence of stronger feelings and more unconscious material.... This experience may be welcomed, may induce near-panic, or may be rejected out of hand. In the final drawing, some people return with relief to their stereotyped pattern; others continue to exercise their new-found freedom; and still others show that they have integrated the new experience even though they choose to use a more deliberate, controlled approach, as in the first drawing. (p. 386)

Many of the early debates about the merits of Naumburg's approach versus Kramer's were loud and long with adherents choosing one or the other. In the 1980s, art therapists began to see the benefit in being able to use either approach depending on the patient's need. Ulman stated that she herself switched between art psychotherapy and art as therapy Although she became an art therapist because of her involvement in art she emphasized that knowing the two poles of the field as defined by Naumburg and Kramer permitted some flexibility in actual clinical work:

I recognize the validity of these two applications of psychoanalytic theory to art therapy practice. Art psychotherapy and art as therapy can exist side by side in the same room at the same time, or in the work of the same therapist at different times. In my own life as a clinician I moved between the two, using art as therapy where I could and shifting to art psychotherapy where the situation seemed to call for it. (Ulman, 1987, p. 286)

Hanna Yaxa Kwiatkowska:
The Invention of Family Art Therapy

Hanna Yaxa Kwiatkowska[12] worked at St. Elizabeths Hospital, a federal facility in Washington, DC, from 1950 to 1958, where she designed her own art therapy programs. During that time she met Frieda Fromm-Reichmann, an encounter which led to her acquiring a position at the National Institute of Mental Health (NIMH) where she stayed for the next 14 years.

She was influenced by a marriage of psychoanalytic theory and the dynamically oriented art therapy approach of Margaret Naumburg. This she combined with the developing body of work by family systems theorists such as Nathan Ackerman, Murray Bowen, Jay Haley, Virginia Satir, and Lyman C. Wynne, among others (Kwiatkowska, 1978, pp. xi–xii). She stressed that artwork done by the family was a means of uncovering unconscious processes and family patterns. But above all, she emphasized a careful, scientifically based approach to her research. "The image itself seems to be the most eloquent spokesman for the inner human experience.... However, I also understood the danger of relying solely on subjective reaction in building any solid theoretical foundation" (p. 215). Consequently, she laid out specific procedures for administering family art evaluations and wrote a manual for rating the pictures (pp. 234–266).

In describing the "particular advantage" of art therapy for families Kwiatkowska said:

> Despite all the vagueness of the family's verbal interpretation of their artwork, that work remains in evidence. Unlike words, it is not evanescent. Therefore it may become a stepping stone toward communication with the family across the curtain of their distortion and denial of meaning. Although work with schizophrenic patients and their families is an unusually taxing and draining experience, the use of art material presents some unique values which help in the arduous communication with these families. (p. 81)

The goal of family art therapy is to uncover unconscious material, to clarify roles within the family system, to promote family communication, and in the case of adjunctive art therapy, to support verbal therapy. This was possible because "the family art therapy session reproduces to a degree the habitual transactions of the family's everyday life" (p. 78).

The role of interpretation is to aid the family members in uncovering symbolic meaning in the art. In the early sessions the family interprets their own artwork. In later ones, the therapists offered their interpretations as well. Kwiatkowska stressed, "Interpretations by the therapists are made only when the family is well engaged in therapy, but even then we try to hear the family's reactions to their and other's pictures first" (p. 28).

Kwiatkowska's family art therapy developed from her work with individual patients and NIMH's emphasis on studying family relations. Due to the research focus of NIMH, she conducted three different types of sessions—family art therapy as the primary mode of treatment, adjunctive family art therapy, and family art evaluations. In all three types of treatment,

> the families' spontaneous art productions were intended to help family members and therapists to better understand the problems in the family, to clarify family members' roles and perceptions of each other, and to constitute a therapeutically useful mode of expression and communication. (p. 8)

The specific tasks[13] for the family art evaluation evolved out of themes which were commonly drawn. This evaluation shares some features with the Ulman Personality Assessment Procedure, especially the arrangement of the tasks in a specific sequence and the use of the scribble which Kwiatkowska asked the family to do both as individuals and as a group. When family art therapy was the primary means of therapy Kwiatkowska generally did not give specific directives but did gradually introduce and repeat the evaluation procedures (p. 140). In a family art evaluation, which Kwiatkowska did in a single session of $1^1/_2$ to 2 hours, she was assisted by a "participant observer" (p. 84) who recorded notes on family interactions and the dynamics of the session. The art therapist provided paper, easels, and semi-hard pastels for this session.

Kwiatkowska espoused active participation of the cotherapists in doing art themselves and honesty in their relationship to the family.

The open expression of the therapists' feeling in pictures portraying their own immediate reactions prompts the family to see more commitment by the therapists. They cease to be the silent impersonal observers who scrutinize and watch. They become part of the family's experience, persons who express their feelings just as they encourage the family to do. Therefore, they can be trusted more easily. (p. 13)

She stressed the importance of clarity in the cotherapists' relationship. Also, she believed it very important for the art therapist to avoid enchantment with or partiality toward a particularly talented family member as this could negatively affect the therapeutic relationship as a whole (p. 27).

When family art therapy was used as an adjunct to conjoint verbal therapy one of the therapists became the art therapist's cotherapist. The art therapist observed as many verbal therapy sessions as possible in order to promote integration of both therapeutic experiences. Usually, the adjunctive art therapy and verbal therapy sessions were held back-to-back with the order of the sessions having a specific effect:

> If family art therapy came first, much material was projected through the art productions that could be further explored in the conjoint family verbal therapy session that followed. If the sequence was reversed, the art therapy provided closure, giving the family an opportunity to express in their pictures emotions stirred in the preceding therapeutic hour. (p. 10)

In talking about the pictures Kwiatkowska followed "up to a point, the general principles of group art therapy" (p. 28). She had a certain approach to inviting others to talk by wondering what the family's reactions were to the pictures and by avoiding direct questions which provoked withdrawal or superficial responses. She found the verbal exchange "to be most therapeutically fruitful when it is stimulated by and directly connected with the pictures" (p. 137). If the art from previous sessions had not been adequately discussed she discouraged making additional pictures.

The family members were asked to give written titles to their artwork:

> The title seems to give some kind of closure to what is graphically expressed; I have found it useful and revealing in many ways. The title may add meaning to a crude design; it may have no connection with what has been drawn; it may have an idiosyncratic connection with the picture; or it may be quite literal, adding nothing. The variety of titles used by different family members, when they have been asked to draw a picture of their family, serves a useful purpose. Titles such as "Family," "My Family," "A Happy Family," "A Mixed-up Family," "People," and "Us" may become the springboard for an animated discussion of how differently the family is viewed by its individual members. (p. 31)

THE NEXT GENERATION

Myra F. Levick:
Art & Defense Mechanisms

Myra Levick obtained a Bachelor of Fine Arts degree from Moore College of Art in Philadelphia. In 1963, she went to work at an inpatient unit for adults at Albert Einstein Medical Center, Northern Division, in Philadelphia. Her title was "art therapist." It was at the clinic that she received training in psychoanalytic theory. In developing an understanding of art therapy, she relied heavily on the writings of Margaret Naumburg, Edith Kramer, and others. During this time at Einstein, she received her master's degree in educational psychology from Temple University.

Levick developed the master's art therapy program at Hahnemann Medical College and Hospital. Levick continued to broaden her understanding of psychology through her studies of family and group psychotherapy. She maintained a private practice and her academic position at Hahnemann, where she taught a variety of subjects. In 1981, Levick received her doctorate in child development from Bryn Mawr College. She is known for her scholarly articles (Levick, 1973, 1983b; Levick,

Goldman, & Fink, 1967; Fink, Goldman, & Levick, 1967), chapters (1981), and two books (1983a, 1986).

Levick believed that psychoanalytic theory was essential in training art therapists to work with a variety of populations, and her own particular interests centered on the ego mechanisms of defense in terms of adaptive and maladaptive behavior patterns. She was also interested in developmental stages, how unresolved conflict led to fixations in these stages, and how these elements are manifested in the drawings of children and adults.

> As the pieces begin to fall into place and complete the 'picture,' they demonstrate that defense mechanisms and intelligence (a function of the conflict-free sphere of the ego), as manifested in spontaneous or directed drawings of children and adults, provide significant information regarding an individual's capacity for adaptation to reality. (Levick, 1983a, p. xvi)

In addition, other information can be found in the pictures:

> Individuals draw in different ways, which reflect their personality traits. Just as someone may be a casual or relaxed housekeeper, someone may draw in a loose, sketchy way. This is not to be confused with regression, which as a defense, is different from one's habitual work habits. (p. 164)

In *Mommy, Daddy, Look What I'm Saying*, Levick states that "anything created by someone—a drawing, a painting, a piece of sculpture—is a nonverbal message from the creator about the inner self and that artist's world" (Levick, 1986, p. 29). Free, undirected drawings and associations are elicited and used to gain a better understanding of areas of conflict. Levick also stresses the validity of both the "art as therapy" and "art in therapy" approaches. While she was working in a hospital setting, she realized the value of the creative process as a means to reduce patients' anxiety without the need to talk about or uncover unconscious material in their drawings.

> Although I was trained in a psychoanalytically oriented milieu, years of experience as a therapist and educator have demonstrated that the most valid goal is that which is consistent with the needs of the patient/client regardless of theoretical orientation. (Levick, 1983a, p. 9)

At Albert Einstein Medical Center, Levick worked adjunctively with other therapists. She states that at different points in treatment, different forms of psychotherapy may take center stage, and others may move from central to an adjunctive position. This all depends on the patient's needs. However, "[art therapy] even when used in conjunction with other psychotherapies, contributes to the therapeutic process beyond that which is generally attributed to an adjunctive therapy" (p. 15).

According to Levick, there are many goals in therapy. However, two of the main goals are to create a therapeutic relationship and to help heal emotional stress. "For all patients/clients, art therapy—a non-verbal form of communication—provides a way to gain distance from disturbing thoughts and feelings" (p. 11). For some patients, the goals are to provide a means for strengthening ego functions and developing impulse control. For others, the goals are to aid in interpersonal relations or to provide a cathartic experience.

Levick points out that it is impossible for an art therapist, regardless of training, to make valid interpretations without direct observation and the client's interpretation. She will offer her own interpretations, but the main focus is centered on the client's. "More recent proponents of Naumburg's original premise believe that the patient's artistic production, like the dream brought to the analyst, cannot be interpreted without the patient's associations" (p. 8).

Levick advocates the necessity of developing skill in therapeutic techniques in order to establish a therapeutic relationship. The art therapist must have experience with all art media in order to carry out varied treatment goals. "The art therapist offers the patient clarifications, connections, confrontations, and interpretations depending on the patient's capacity to handle the material being expressed" (Levick, 1975c, p. 94).

In an early paper, Levick investigated how transference and countertransference were manifested in art (Levick, 1975b). She agreed with Naumburg that art therapy permitted the working through of transference feelings and, therefore, aided in dealing with resistance to therapy.

> For those dynamically oriented art therapists, the goal is to allow the transference relationship to develop so that through the patients' associations to their spontaneous drawings, insights into conflictual areas of the psyche may be uncovered. In the process of making verbal what was non-verbal, conscious what was unconscious, the art psychotherapist makes connections and clarifications in an effort to help the patient interpret his/her own symbolic images. (Levick, 1983a, p. 9)

Levick discusses the importance of the client's talking about the art in certain situations and then states that this is not necessary in others. This is consistent with her reliance on different approaches depending on the client's needs. "Art therapy can provide an activity that may alleviate anxiety. In this art activity, verbalization may not be elicited and is, in fact, not necessary. Gratification is obtained from the act of participating in the creative process" (p. 12).

It is clear that Levick understands the importance of the aesthetic value of the artwork, but does not depend upon it to the same degree as Kramer. She uses artwork as a means for the client to communicate unconscious material to the art therapist.

Helen Landgarten: Clinical Art Therapy

On the East Coast, the first art therapists found jobs in psychiatric hospitals where they functioned as part of the treatment team, providing treatment which was adjunctive to that of the psychiatrist. The 1970s and 1980s saw the development of art therapists with the training and opportunities to act as a special kind of psychotherapist equivalent to social workers, psychologists, and marriage and family therapists, but with additional expertise in nonverbal processes. Art therapists trained in this way were often able to find employment as primary practitioners, thus expanding the identity and influence of art therapy as a mental health discipline. Helen Landgarten has been a major influence in this trend and in the current training and definition of art psychotherapists.

Clinical Art Therapy: A Comprehensive Guide (Landgarten, 1981) provides a model of practice that includes a wide age range and a variety of settings including outpatient clinics, psychiatric hospitals, and rehabilitation centers. The book is also explicit in its definition of an art therapist as a psychotherapist with special tools and abilities capable of functioning as a primary care clinician. She coined the term "clinical art therapy" and used it to define her master's training program.

Helen Landgarten grew up in Detroit and moved to California after she married. After raising two children, she returned to school in her forties, earned her Bachelor of Fine Arts, and did graduate work in painting, sculpting, and printmaking at the University of California at Los Angeles (UCLA). Landgarten recalls:

> Somewhere along the line I decided painting wasn't enough for me, that I wanted to work in the community. I had gone through a sensitivity training course and felt I had two talents, as an artist and as a therapist. I decided I wanted to combine the two. I did some work in a county hospital adolescent unit. They called it art therapy. (1975)

As a psychologically oriented artist, Landgarten began in the mid-1960s to seek ways to merge creativity in art and psychodynamic theory as therapy for the mentally ill. This thrust grew out of her experimental work in therapeutically and psychologically oriented art education with geriatric clients in a community center in 1964, and her later work on an inpatient unit at Los Angeles County/USC Hospital.

In 1968, Landgarten became an art therapist in the Department of Psychiatry in the Family, Child Division, Mt. Sinai Medical Center in Los Angeles. (This later became the Thalians Community Mental Health Center of Cedars-Sinai Hospital.) She recalls:

> I gave a presentation at Cedars-Sinai and presented what I would like to do at the hospital. The agreement was that they would give me a group of adolescents and if, at the end of six weeks, they liked what I did, they would hire me and they did. (1975)

Landgarten became the Director of Art Psychotherapy there under the auspices of Dr. Saul Brown, a psychiatrist and noted family therapist. In addition, she trained at the Mt. Sinai outpatient clinic as an art therapy clinician, not only providing adjunctive therapy but carrying full case responsibility. Landgarten defines her orientation as that of an art psychotherapist:

> The word "therapist" is important [in my work]. I don't see it as recreation therapy or as adjunctive. I am the primary therapist. Most art therapists are not art psychotherapists. I make a distinction between therapeutic art and art psychotherapy. (1975)

In 1973, she started the master's program in clinical art therapy at Immaculate Heart College, which moved in 1980 to Loyola Marymount University. She retired from Loyola in 1987. She continued to work at Thalians as Coordinator of Art Psychotherapy, developing a department with five art psychotherapists, until her retirement in 1991.

Landgarten's contributions were immensely important to the expansion of art therapy on the West Coast and to the recognition of a "clinical art therapy" approach. Her second book, *Family Art Psychotherapy*, was published in 1987. *Adult Art Psychotherapy: Issues and Applications,* edited with Darcy Lubbers, was published in 1991.[14] Landgarten's particular interest and contributions are in family art therapy.

Landgarten's theoretical base is psychodynamic (neo-Freudian) in that she adheres to Freud's definition of personality composed of the id, ego, and super-ego. In her family work, she integrates the psychodynamic theory of personality with the here-and-now approach of family systems theorists, principally Bowen, Ackerman, Minuchin, Whitaker, Bell, Haley, Satir, and others. To this base she adds the use of flexible and eclectic behavioral and problem-solving techniques. She believes, "It is...important that art psychotherapy be understood as a psychotherapeutic technique, syntonic with all existing family therapy theories" (Landgarten, 1987, p. xix).

Landgarten takes a directed approach to art therapy which is practical and goal-oriented. The art therapist works with the family to achieve a more effective level of functioning by first upsetting "the old balance" and helping to "organize a more satisfying one.... The *invading device is the art directive, which contains the appropriate media and is clinically sound....* [The directive is] *dictated by the dynamics of each session with consideration to short- and long-term goals*" (p. 5, emphasis in the original).

The goals of therapy vary depending on whether the therapy involves an individual, a family, or a group. Individual goals might be gaining psychological awareness, reality-testing, problem-solving, revealing unconscious material, catharsis, working through conflicts, and/or separation/individuation. Family therapy goals might be the resolution of the presenting problem and the facilitation of family tasks which parallel the developmental phases in the family life cycle. Group therapy goals are dependent upon the makeup of the group.

Landgarten's approach defines the art therapist as the primary therapist. The therapist takes an active role as an agent of change in the here-and-now by the use of goal-oriented art directives. She sees the therapist's role as intruding on the family system in an attempt to upset the homeostasis and to give support to a restructured family system. It is also the therapist's role to educate patients to record thoughts, emotions, and associations which relate to their artwork; to encourage clients to understand the correlation between their artwork and themselves; to provide insightful feedback; and to give clear art directives around relevant issues. The therapist must also be vigilant for overt and covert messages in the artwork and the art-making process. "The family art therapist must be creative in two areas simultaneously; while being psychologically attuned to the participants, he or she must make an immediate decision about the appropriate art task which shall serve a therapeutic purpose" (p. 281).

Understanding the "metaphoric blueprint concept" (which is Landgarten's term for the relationship of artwork to the client or family) "has a positive effect as it tends to hasten a positive transference which is especially necessary for family therapy" (p. 5).

The client's own interpretation of his/her artwork is paramount, although other interpretations are possible based on the therapist's frame(s) of reference. Landgarten is a strong proponent of understanding personal symbolism, which may shift not only from individual to individual, but also within the individual from stage to stage within the life cycle. The therapist provides insightful feedback, being cautious of the client's ability and readiness to receive such feedback. She does not seek universal symbols.

Talking aids in uncovering unconscious material as well as adding to a patient's ownership and responsibility for his/her own work in therapy. Making art and talking about it is done in each art therapy session: first, the art directive is given and the art is created, and then, the client and the therapist discuss and process the art. Landgarten believes that

Before the session ends, ...it is important for therapists to state their observations, in order to give support to the reality of the family process. The clinician's verbalized interactional assessment gains credibility through the visual proof of the product itself. The artwork is always referred to as the source for the psychotherapist's insight to lessen omnipotent fantasies about the therapist within the transference phenomenon. (p. 16)

The art process, rather than the aesthetic value of the artwork, is the focus. If concerns about performance are mentioned, the therapist offers assurance by declaring that "the art, per se, is unimportant since there are no expectations either about the way in which the art is created or about the end product itself" (p. 14). The content of the artwork serves Landgarten as an external portrayal of intrapsychic communication, as a record of the therapeutic process, and as a catalyst for change.

> The value of the art task is threefold: the *process* as a diagnostic, interactional, and rehearsal tool; the *contents* as a means of portraying unconscious and conscious communication; and the *product* as lasting evidence of the group's dynamics. (p. 5, emphasis in the original)

Arthur Robbins:
An Object Relations Approach

Arthur Robbins is Professor of Art Therapy at Pratt Institute in Brooklyn and the Director of the Institute for Expressive Analysis in New York City. A faculty member of the National Psychological Association for

Psychoanalysis, he also maintains a private practice of art therapy and psychoanalysis in New York City.

Robbins has contributed four books to the field: *Creative Art Therapy* (Robbins & Sibley, 1976), *Expressive Therapies* (1980), *The Artist as Therapist* (1987a), and *The Psychoaesthetic Experience* (1989).

Robbins believes that to be maximally effective in psychoanalytic psychotherapy, the exploration of the common properties and the binding of art and science are necessary. During a sculpture class, Robbins first became aware of the parallels between the creative and therapeutic processes (Robbins, 1987a, p. 12) and that "the aesthetic and therapeutic processes themselves reflect the same integration of fusion and separateness" (p. 22). He felt that aesthetics was a form of giving life to the inanimate and the making of statements of who one is; symbols become a codification and an organization of one's self.

Robbins' theoretical stance comes from object relations theory: "It is these early internalized relationships with their effect on one's current reality which form the core of object relations theory as I use it in my practice" (Robbins, 1987b, p. 65). Robbins stresses that when he speaks of object relations theory he is "not referring to one unified theory" but that the "term reflects my own distillation from a body of theory, itself derived from classical psychoanalytic theory" (p. 66). Object relations theory, as summarized by Robbins,

> presents an organized structure clarifying the subtle and complex interrelationships of self and other that we all carry within us. Other, or "object," refers to the who and the what in which we invest our libidinal energy. By libidinal energy I refer to the life force in an individual that is partly sexual and partly aggressive but is more than either. It is the fuel that motivates each of us to reach out and invest in the world around us. (Robbins, 1987a, p. 24)

According to Robbins, relationships are characterized by various energy systems forming the shape and space around us; each system has levels of openness or closure, completeness or incompleteness.

Two key constructs he uses from other writers are Winnicott's concept of the "holding environment" (Winnicott, 1971) and Mahler's specific stages of psychological separation/individuation (Mahler, Pine, & Bergman, 1975). The holding environment is "that space between patient and therapist in which we complement or mirror our patient's inner representational world" (Robbins, 1987a, p. 61). This fosters ego growth and facilitates reconnection to primary creativity. The representations of both the therapist's and the patient's pasts

> express themselves ... as energy sensation, color, rhythm, volume, weight. Slowly, with the artwork and therapist's holding, organizing, reflecting back the patient's internal pathological state, the patient is given the chance to play with unresolved polarities and representations to find new integrations and solutions. (p. 27)

Art materials can be used "to promote an ever adapting holding environment sensitive to the patient's changing levels of ego integration, defenses, resistances, object representations, and the like" (p. 104).

> In essence, the therapist creates a holding environment in which empathy is the basis of communication..... [A]s in a work of art, the nature of empathy is metaphorical and symbolic, its messages organized through visual, kinesthetic, auditory, or verbal levels, singly or in combination. (p. 27)

Knowing Mahler's developmental stages makes it possible to work "with a patient who has failed to navigate successfully these very early developmental crises, [for] the task of treatment becomes one of building rather than uncovering" (p. 26). According to Mahler, the therapist becomes the lost object of the patient and offers part of his/her organizing ego.

Through the creative process the patient is able to re-create various representations of inner and outer worlds. Artwork acts as an organizer, mirroring internal object relations and any associated defenses and/or developmental problems. Art therapy promotes delving into levels of perceptual organization which allows a shifting of energy patterns from negative to positive awareness and enactment.

> Art therapy, then, strives to promote new levels of perceptual organization that involves shifts in energy patterns. The art form offers an added means for working with splits and polarities and integrating them into new wholes. The representations from our past are expressed through image and symbol and expand the boundaries of objective reality.... Being nonverbal in nature, these symbols and images are often difficult to express clearly in verbal form and therefore lend themselves well to the medium of art. (Robbins, 1987b, p. 68)

The goal of therapy is for the patient's life space to expand so there is a richer symbolic imaginative life that can lead to true creativity. Therapeutic goals are not exclusively directed toward uncovering unconscious material, but differ according to the personality disorder of the patient.

> In therapy, patients and therapists alike are engaged in finding the artists within themselves. The therapeutic process for patients is an ongoing struggle to discover true inner representations and symbols and then give them form in terms of developing richer, more congruent living realities. (Robbins, 1987a, p. 21)

The therapist needs to understand the developmental level of the patient and must reflect upon the various parts of him/herself which may relate to some of the internal representations of the patient. A bridge is created between patient and therapist. The therapist focuses awareness on his/her feelings and internalized objects and on the client's so that they can be molded into communication. In this manner, the intangible can become explicit. For his part, Robbins says:

> I remain open but controlled, spontaneous but not wild.... Clearly, interpretation in this sense involves more than making the unconscious conscious or connecting past and present. It gives shape and form to the myriad relationships being played out in the psychological space between therapist and patient as their internalized objects make contact and react to one another. (Robbins, 1989, p. 231)

Talking clarifies and connects the world of the inner experience to the outer world of words. Words are used syntonically with the patient's strengths and defense mechanisms as it takes time for the artworks' subtle integration to occur and then the complex structure of words becomes available. Depending on the situation, art sometimes supports, contradicts, or enlarges the verbal associations In Robbins' art therapy, talking seems to take an important, but complementary, role to the art expression. "Changing art expression into poetic metaphor serves as a transition to the world of words and helps make sense of the truism that although verbal material is strongly connected to reality, not all of reality is encompassed by words" (Robbins, 1987a, p. 36).

The artwork is a safe container for transference issues which are defined by the early development of object relationships. These issues are reconstructed and resolved in the artwork. Early object relations are frequently colored with loss, annihilation, pain, and love. But,

> the real relationship between patient and therapist becomes every bit as important as the transference, as the therapist opens himself up and taps the various parts of himself that may mirror, complement, or confront the various representations of the patient. (p. 27)

Robbins gives specific meaning to aesthetics which he says refers "to making the inanimate animate, giving form to diffuse energy or ideas, breathing life to sterile communication" (p. 22). As integration takes place and symbolic forms emerge to communicate a larger meaning, the artwork approaches the level of aesthetic communication. The aesthetic value is not in defensive artistic artwork, but in "an aesthetic integration of symbolic form in the ongoing identity process" (p. 23).

> In art therapy ... we are constantly working to make aesthetic expression a complement to self-expression in one's relationship with others. In that process, the art therapist works with an individual's character defenses and slowly helps him to digest emotionally the full impact of the symbolic communications so that there is a real awareness of what is being said in symbolic form and of how the client can manifest that in his ongoing relationships with others. That implies a considerable working through, which becomes the province of the art therapist. (p. 23)

As for the combination of art and therapy, Robbins maintains that

> As art therapists, our skills in integrating all this offer a special and powerful dimension to a therapeutic team. Our challenge will be one of utilizing these concepts from

psychiatry and psychoanalysis, while maintaining the visions and perceptions we have as artists. (p. 74)

Judith Rubin:
A Psychoanalytic Approach to Art Therapy

Judith Rubin realized the emotional impact of the art process at age seventeen when a friend died in a senseless accident. Making art became a "way of coping with trauma too difficult to assimilate.... It did not take away the hurt and the ache, but it helped release some of the rage, and gave form to a multiplicity of feelings and wishes" (Rubin, 1978, p. 10).

Rubin received a bachelor's in art from Wellesley College, a master's in education from the Harvard Graduate School of Education and a doctorate in counselling from the University of Pittsburgh. She has been part of the Psychoanalysis Training Program at the Pittsburgh Psychoanalytic Institute, co-director of the Creative and Expressive Arts Therapy Program at Western Psychiatric Institute and Clinic, and assistant professor of Child Psychiatry and Health Related Professions at the University of Pittsburgh. She was the "Art Lady" on the television show "Misterogers' Neighborhood." Rubin is a former President and an Honorary Life Member of the American Art Therapy Association. She has worked with children who have schizophrenia and those who have physical disabilities.

Rubin emphasizes the importance of discovering the early origins of psychological disturbance and of using a developmental frame of reference to understand both the person and the art. Accordingly, she is interested in the theories which were derived from Freud's, including ego psychology, object relations, and self-psychology. However, her theoretical base is fundamentally psychoanalytic (Rubin, 1987b, p. 12). She stresses that in psychoanalytic therapy:

> The therapist helps the patient to understand and gain control over maladaptive patterns of thought and behavior by questions, clarifications, confrontations, and other forms of intervention—especially interpretations in which connections are made explicit.... [Goals are] uncovering repressed material...and helping the patient gain insight into the meaning of his behavior.... I find the use of art in an insight-oriented approach to be the most powerful and exciting kind of art therapy for myself, as well as for most of my patients. (p. 12)

Rubin sees the releasing of the unconscious in symbolic form by encouraging free associations and free expression as the optimal route to repressed material. Through the creative process art gives form to that which is feared or repressed (unconscious), which allows for integration and synthesis by organizing thought and action. Rubin devotes considerable discussion to the "framework for freedom" (Rubin, 1978, Chapter 1) which the art therapist provides. She stresses that the "order in creative activity" (p. 21) permits an individual to experience psychological freedom. The art therapist or any "provider of art...must make possible a productive and integrated relationship between the two" (p. 22).

The therapist must know the history of the person in order to establish the most meaningful therapeutic encounter:

> When development goes awry at any point in a person's life, whether the disability is inborn or acquired as the result of some physical stress, then subsequent development is necessarily affected. In order to not only name the problem but to understand its etiology, one must know its historical origins. Only with this kind of underpinning can a therapist know how to best help a patient. (Rubin, 1984, pp. 41–42)

Earlier, when writing about her work with children, Rubin said:

> While it is not essential to have a detailed understanding of development and psychodynamics in order to provide good, creative, broadly "therapeutic" art experiences...it is

my conviction that the more one understands, the more one can help. With the very disturbed child, understanding is essential. (Rubin, 1978, p. 75)

The therapist provides a predictable environment, with continuity, security, limits, and regulation of boundaries. "The artistry of good therapy lies in being flexible within certain guidelines, reflecting an image of freedom with order and energy with control" (Rubin, 1984, p. 53).

Therapy is a partnership based on a therapeutic working alliance. The therapist adapts a neutral stance enabling the patient to project feelings and ideas reflecting unresolved conflicts. "An important tool in this kind of treatment is the transference: the symbolic ways in which the patient perceives and responds to the therapist. It helps both participants to identify distorted perceptions based on unresolved conflicts from the past" (Rubin, 1987b, p. 12).

While the art therapist in his encounter with a client is in many ways a very real person, there are symbolic aspects of the role which are important.... In one sense, these refer to the distorted symbolic ways—the transference—in which the relationship is experienced by the client(s). In another sense, they refer to the particular activities of the art therapist, which themselves carry symbolic meanings. The two are related, for the behaviors of the art therapist inevitably influence the kind of transference which develops, as well as its understanding and use as a vehicle for change.

The concept of transference is a useful one for an art therapist to know, and is quite congenial, for it is simply an extension of the human sphere of what is already suspected about the meaning of artistic symbols. (Rubin, 1978, p. 256)

The art therapist is facilitator, provider, and nurturer (p. 257) to the patient, encouraging and stimulating conditions for growth. But Rubin cautions, "Adults have different reasons for going into service professions, and a not-uncommon motivation is one's own concerns about nurturance.... It is understandable that one might identify with the hurt and needy child, and in so doing feel compelled to give" (p. 75).

But just as there are "giving" and "nurturing" aspects of the transference feelings there are negative ones too. Rubin points out that the art therapist may be perceived as a voyeur, a seducer, a prober, or other dangerous person as she carries out her customary role (p. 257).

As treatment begins, it is essential, according to Rubin, to concentrate on enhancing the comfort level of the patient by being more supportive, less confrontive, and establishing expectations for sessions. Both nonverbal and verbal behavior are carefully observed.

A therapist cannot work with a patient over any substantial period of time without establishing some kind of working relationship... art therapists are in a rather favorable position in the establishment of an alliance with patients, since what we offer is not only ourselves but our modality as well. In a sense, then the patient forms an alliance over time with both the therapist and the creative process. (Rubin, 1984, p. 54)

Child Art Therapy (1978) presents Rubin's work with individuals, families, and groups in a clinic setting and with children in the community. Rubin is particularly persuasive in her descriptions of the benefits of art therapy with blind and multiply-disabled children:

The use of art materials like clay as fantasied replacements, additions, or perhaps protectors is also common with the blind.... it seemed to be a way of compensating in fantasy for the missing body part or function, and may also have served as protection against the ever-present threat of further injury. (Rubin, 1978, pp. 121-122)

Rubin admits that "working with blind and otherwise handicapped children in therapy has never been easy for me, but it has always been both a challenge and a powerful learning experience" (p. 124). She has produced a movie about her work with this population entitled "We'll Show You What We're Gonna Do!" (1972).

Addressing her use of theory, Rubin states:

> In the course of my own development, I have read, studied, and worked with different theoretical perspectives, and have usually found in each one or more concepts relevant to the work I do.
>
> Until quite recently, I thought that the solution to my problem [of formulating a theoretical orientation] would be a kind of patchwork—a mosaic or collage of different ideas from different theories—which together would account for what seems to happen in art therapy.... What now seems more probable is that a theory about art therapy will have to emerge from art therapy itself. It will no doubt partake of elements of other perspectives, but it will need to have its own inner integrity in terms of the creative process of which it consists. (Rubin, 1978, p. 18)

In *The Art of Art Therapy* (1984) Rubin explores how to think about doing art therapy and says that "in a way, the whole book is an attempt to describe what goes into making a good art therapist" (p. vi). In her careful look at the various facets of art therapy, Rubin has added immeasurably to the type of information necessary for a specific theory of art therapy to grow. However, while she relied primarily on her understanding of psychoanalytic theory in her first book, Rubin wrote "I do not feel ready to develop and articulate a definitive theoretical statement about art as, in, or for therapy" (1978, p. 19).

In the meantime, the number of new psychological theories and corresponding therapeutic techniques increased dramatically. In *Approaches to Art Therapy* (1987a) Rubin solicited chapters by art therapists representing some of these different theoretical bents. Her broad survey presents a map of the field and its boundaries which encompasses considerably more than psychoanalytic theory. In her conclusion to this work, Rubin points out the problems art therapists have had in deciding which theoretical approach provided the best fit with what they do. But, she thinks, "all of the contributors seem to agree on at least two things: (1) the importance of the image and (2) the complexity of both person and process in art therapy. And whatever the relative emphasis on art and therapy in any author's conception, all include a consideration of both" (Rubin, 1987c, p. 324). In presenting such a collective work she had hoped to "multiply the number of 'listening and looking perspectives' potentially available to each clinician, so that he or she can receive, perceive, and conceive as well as possible when dealing with different patients at different times" (p. 319).

ALTERNATIVE PERSPECTIVES

Although the prevailing model for art therapy practice and theory, like the seminal works of Naumburg and Kramer, is based on a psychoanalytic/psychodynamic premise, other points of view have their followers. This section addresses what we consider to be the most important alternative perspectives.

Mala Betensky:
Phenomenology & Art Therapy

In 1973, Mala Betensky wrote *Self-Discovery Through Self-Expression* which presented a theoretical approach different in philosophy, goals, and technique from the prevailing models which were psychoanalytically and psychodynamically based. Despite offering a compelling counter theory, Betensky's model has not been widely adopted. We speculate that this may be due in part to her lack of a permanent base in an academic training program in the United States which would provide continuous contact with new generations of art therapists. In addition, the prevailing psychoanalytic *Zeitgeist* of the profession may have moderated against her point of view.

Betensky is a clinical psychologist and art therapist in private practice in Washington, DC. She lectures in the United States and Israel and is affiliated with Haifa University (in the Department of Expressive Therapies) and Yelin College in Israel. She earned doctorates from the New School for Social Research in both sociology and psychology and has done artwork in ceramic sculpture and woodworking. Betensky distinguished herself by being the first person to publish a book with in-depth case studies using art therapy as the primary psychotherapy (1973). She is one of only two "first generation" art therapy pioneers who did not subscribe to a psychoanalytic point of view.[15]

Betensky describes her theoretical base as an open system with three major components: phenomenology (specifically, phenomenological psychology), tenets of Gestalt psychology, and studies of art, especially the writings of artists.

Phenomenology is the study of events and happenings in their own right rather than from the point of view of inferred causes. The phenomenologist attempts to come as close to the lived experience of the phenomenon as possible. Betensky's philosophy also reflects humanistic thought in that developing the conscious self is the unifying theme. The experience of coming to know oneself (awareness of self, integrating self, and self-actualization) is the essence of the approach. Personal growth is stressed (rather than focusing on unconscious conflicts); a positive view of human nature and human potential is a key element of phenomenological psychology.

> While trait theory of personality assigns the individual into a diagnostic category and predicts his future behavior, and the psychodynamic personality model leans on the unconscious, both theories neglect the rich and illuminating variety of states of the conscious, quite potent in relation to the human ability to change. (Betensky, 1973, p. 336)

According to Betensky, Gestalt theory and the concepts of phenomenology are very similar to each other. The "whole" quality of the phenomenon (for instance, art expression) or the Gestalt is important. What makes a whole are the components that are parts of the structure. Major structural components of art are line, shape, and color which can be explored in therapy. The relationship of other art structures such as hues, foreground, background, location on the page, shading, and perspective can also be examined. The relationship of these structures to each other is the answer to what makes a whole.

Betensky emphasizes that the literature and scientific research regarding the structure of art written prior to the time of Freud has been influential in her work. She specifically mentions William James's work on the stream of consciousness and Karl Jaspers' writings on hypnosis and creativity

For Betensky, the person is born into the world and must relate to it. When the patient comes to art therapy he/she is in an intermediate position between being lost and imprisoned by the world and a need to discover the self again in the world. The person is organized within a series of unities (body and mind, emotions and thought). A lack of unity creates a disturbance and the client needs help in becoming aware of this in order to move toward a more unified self. Drawing restores bits of the authentic self. Three forces in the art therapy process are described: visual perception (seeing the art), cognitive perception (talking about the art), and emotion (feeling associated with the art).

> I combined the art therapy technique with clinical findings, psychological insights, and social considerations to help the individual discover his authentic self. One of the characteristics of a disturbed person is that he is not always conscious of his own behavior. When an individual experiences himself through art, he sometimes manages to restore his stream of awareness. This is an act of self discovery....

> This therapy was present oriented...[and] was also change oriented. (Betensky, 1973, p. xi)

During an art therapy session Betensky allows the patient to engage freely with art materials. When the artwork is complete she asks the patient to place it on the wall (visual display), to step back from the drawing (distancing), and to look at the whole picture from corner to corner, and from top to bottom (intentional looking). She then uses simple questions to guide the patient's seeing. She believes it is more effective to talk about the relationship of the specific structural components of the art than about the content of the image per se. She views such relationships as metaphors for human relationships and that they carry, promote, and convey feelings by their very nature. Once visual relationships are established, patterns of awareness emerge.

Art therapy is used as a vehicle for communication and a method of expressing the self—from the preverbal to the verbal, from the implicit to the explicit. Through art expression, relationships and patterns emerge which provide the "aha experience," a sudden sense of awareness. From awareness, the individual moves to integrating the experience with real life and taking responsibility for feelings and for change.

[Patients] assume responsibility for their artwork from the start and actively participate in the intellectual and artistic process of working through the difficulties that have arisen in interactions between themselves and others. This is the particular contribution of the phenomenological approach to art expression in therapy—arrived at through artwork and the subsequent treatment of the organization of the art expression—from preintentional functioning to fully intentional living. (Betensky, 1987, p. 165)

Betensky describes the "general outline" of her phenomenological method of art therapy as follows:

Sequence 1: Pre-art play with art materials

               Direct experiencing

Sequence 2: The process of artwork—

               Creating a phenomenon

Sequence 3: Phenomenological intuiting

    Phase 1: Perceiving

           1. Visual display

           2. Distancing

           3. Intentional looking

    Phase 2: What-do-you-see procedure

           1. Phenomenological description

           2. Phenomenological unfolding

Sequence 4: Phenomenological integration (p. 158).

In Betensky's approach,

The therapist's task is to watch the client at work, in addition to giving active guidance or participating in other ways [such as standing with the client to view the art]. It is largely a silent task, but the therapist as participant-observer, is far from being passive. He or she is busy unobtrusively observing the client's facial and bodily expressions of moods and his modes of choosing and using art materials during the creative process. Sensing to what extent the client needs the art therapist's physical closeness or other support is another aspect of the task, and noticing one's own visceral and motional reactions to what the client does is yet another. (Geller, 1980, as summarized in Betensky, 1987, p. 157)

According to Betensky, in art therapy the transference is three-dimensional and happens through the art experience.

When past events were re-experienced through a painting or sculpture, that art production became instrumental in helping the young expressionist specify old, lingering feelings which had originated in the past events, but had been carried in patterns of mechanistic transference into subsequent situations, objectively different from the historical ones. Such lingering feelings carried on a life of their own..., strong enough to block development. (Betensky, 1973, p. 342)

Betensky acknowledges the concept of transference but aims to dilute it by disclosing it to the client. The vehicle of transference is the art material and the artwork. This point of view dictates her position as an active interpersonal therapist. Betensky indicates that the client simultaneously experiences and resolves his/her transference through the art process. "Transference in the form of feelings about parents transferred onto the therapist [is] also treated in art psychotherapy as a vehicle for bringing the past into the present, to reexamine it in the light of the present" (p. 343).

Regarding the role of talking in art therapy, Betensky writes:

> Yes, the phenomenological approach does use speech, because words are expression, just as art is; because consciousness, thought, and speech are one; and because in phenomenology we intend to articulate, and that is the job of words. In this method, however, words have a special role at an appropriate time. (Betensky, 1987, p. 157)

The aesthetic quality of the art is not important. All art is accepted and used as a vehicle for communication. Self-expression through art is the connecting link between the inside and the outside. What has been internal thus finds an outlet and provides a basis for growth.

To Betensky,

> art therapy comes the closest to the fulfillment of the task
> that Heidegger assigned to phenomenology: revealing the
> hidden aspects of man's being as phenomena accessible to
> consciousness and to conscious investigation. Art therapy
> can best achieve this aim phenomenologically by means
> of a free expressive process, with art materials freely cho-
> sen by the client, along with a method in which the client
> views his art production as a phenomenon within a struc-
> tured field of vision. (p. 154)

Janie Rhyne:
The Gestalt Art Experience

Born in Florida, Janie Rhyne earned her bachelor's
degree from Florida State College for Women where she
studied art and psychology. She taught art in inner city
schools in Philadelphia and painted on her own. She has
a master's in art and cultural anthropology and lived in
Mexico, Spain, Germany, and Canada. When she went
back to graduate school, she discovered Gestalt
psychology. Rhyne remembers:

> I was intrigued and excited. For the first time academic
> theoretical psychology came together with what I was do-
> ing in art. I was very excited about it and became increas-
> ingly aware that I had been using Gestalt psychological

principles without even knowing it.... I realized I'd been
doing art therapy but had never called myself an art therapist nor heard of Margaret Naumburg or Edith Kramer.
(Rhyne, 1975)

Rhyne went to San Francisco in the 1960s because of
her interest in the Esalen Institute, one of the centers of
the human potential movement on the Northern California coast, and because of her wish to contact Fritz Perls,
the eminent Gestalt therapist. She trained with Perls for 2
years, ran art groups for children and adults, and saw
private patients. Rhyne lived in the Haight-Ashbury district of San Francisco as the hippie movement began,
flourished, and finally died because of drugs and violence. She introduced a drop-in clinic, "The Off-Ramp,"
and began the Gestalt Therapy Institute of San Francisco
with two other therapists in 1968. Rhyne states:

I was using art with hippies and flower children. Art was a
natural there ... the way I used it was more for process
than product oriented. We worked with a lot of clay and
with the movement of hands ... the clinic also drew very
high caliber psychotherapists. It was very exciting and art
was the important part of it. (1975)

With the encouragement of the humanistic theorist
Abraham Maslow, she took the notes she had kept of her
work and put together a book which was published in

1973 as *The Gestalt Art Experience*. It was also in 1973 that Rhyne began studies for her doctorate in psychology.

Gestalt psychology and Gestalt therapy provide the theoretical base of Rhyne's Gestalt art therapy. Important influences on her thinking were Lewin's field theories of group dynamics and Goldstein's organismic theory, including his belief in the organization, unity, and consistency of the normal person. Pathology is created by the impact of negative environmental stress. Rhyne has been heavily influenced by her mentor Fritz Perls and his wife Laura Perls who based their psychotherapy techniques on Goldstein's theory.

Using a humanistic framework Rhyne views human development as a process of self-awareness and therapy as one way in which blocks to awareness may be removed to allow for natural, innate growth. She sees art within therapy as a powerful vehicle for personality integration and personal development. Rhyne explains:

> Most of us are not allowed to grow up naturally, to learn through experience...we are forced to deny much of what we know to be true about our own nature.... Most of us, by the time we are considered adult and mature, have forgotten how to be ourselves. We remember just enough of what being ourselves feels like to be afraid of it....

Gestaltists offer ways to get through this wall of fear—
we seek ways to recognize what we have hidden away—
and to integrate our disowned parts into our total
personality. (Rhyne, 1973, pp. 3–4)

In combining the use of art with a Gestalt theoretical
approach, Rhyne views art as a metaphor for reality:

[The] presence [of the art] allows us to experience and express immediate perceptions and awareness. We do not
have to talk *about* configurations, figure/ground relationships, dynamic movement, contact/boundaries, coherence
and fragmentation in the abstract; rather we speak *of* these
phenomena in the very act of perceiving and becoming
aware of what is obviously there. (Rhyne, 1987, pp.
172–173, emphasis in the original)

The art then shows a similarity in its structure to that of
human behavior, a concept which is encompassed by the
Gestalt principle of isomorphism. "We contact each other
through the presence of the drawing, seeing the interplay
of lines, shapes and forms within the wholeness of it as
a Gestalt" (p. 173).

Integration of the whole, including becoming conscious of ways in which the client is blocking his or her
own experiencing of the present, and the actualization of
a person's inherent potential are the goals of therapy for
Rhyne. "We are working together with an existential aim

of facilitating the client's awareness that she is responsible for choicemaking and for self-direction in living her own life" (p. 185).

The client makes his/her own interpretation of the relationships within and among the artworks and between the messages in the art and life. "Without pushing for interpretations, we explore the dimensions of the drawing and elaborate its impact through active present experiencing" (p. 173).

The therapist engages in exploration of visual representations, actively perceiving and responding in the therapy session. She helps the person work towards integration of the parts to the whole self in the here-and-now. "Gestalt art therapists work toward activating in all clients their best potential for perceiving in their own visual messages, their needs, and their resources" (p. 187).

The client is encouraged to have direct experiences to resolve any conflict or unfinished business from the past. By predominantly experiencing the conflict rather than just talking about it the patient is able to expand his/her level of awareness and integrate whatever was unknown or fragmented into his/her whole being. "In my work as an art therapist, patients, clients, students and I communicate verbally, of course, but we do so mostly in reference to some representations they have created in non-verbal media" (p. 172).

Rhyne's approach to transference[16] is radically different from those therapists who have a psychoanalytic orientation: "Transference is not encouraged; it is seen as an avoidance of the present-centered, person-to-person relationship" (p. 172). The person is responsible for the course of his/her life, and is encouraged to use one's innate potential for full development and growth. Rhyne believes that no human being can be anything other than subjective in a relationship, thus she enters into a mutual relationship with the client hoping for changes in both of them.

The art product is valued for its relationship to the whole of the client's life and for the awareness and meaning which can be derived from it. Rhyne's definition of art changed from the time she was "artistically snobbish" and "knew what art was." She came to understand that the various approaches to art, from fine art to craft to a mode of self-expression, were not mutually exclusive. She exhorts: "Let's put aside the categorizing that is not relevant to art as personal experience. Let's use art to make us more aware of ourselves as psychic and social beings" (Rhyne, 1973, pp. 98–99).

In speaking of her relationship to the field of art therapy, Rhyne said:

> I didn't even know about it until long after it had started. Most of the people were originally psychoanalytical and [used the] medical model. However, I met a number of these people, specifically Elinor Ulman and Hanna Kwiatkowska, and found that though they claimed to be staunchly psychoanalytical and I claimed to be a staunch Gestaltist, we operate as therapists pretty much the same way. (1975)

During an interview conducted by the Department of History at the University of Louisville Rhyne was asked what she would like to be remembered for. She gave this interesting response: "I would like to be remembered as one who showed you could go on learning even beyond the age of forty...as one who started a Ph.D. program at the age of 60 and can get it by 65" (1975).

Rawley Silver:
A Cognitive Approach

After a career in social work, Rawley Silver became a painter when her children were young. When an accident temporarily deafened her she became interested in deaf children:

I found great pleasure in painting and after the accident began to wonder what my life would have been like if I had been deafened as a child, and what role art played in the education of deaf children. I visited art classes in schools for the deaf and was appalled by what I saw. (Silver, 1985, p. 30)

Silver returned to school to prepare herself to work with the deaf. She earned a doctorate in fine arts and fine arts education from Columbia University in 1961, began her work with children, and soon after published reports on the role of art in intellectual and emotional development. Her work was greeted with hostility:

Some educators of the deaf saw it [art] as a form of manual communication which I had never learned and which was forbidden in most schools for the deaf in the 1960s and early 1970s. The antagonism of those who favored lip-reading and speech toward those who still used sign language was emotional and often personal and bitter. (p. 31)

Silver started working with deaf children and later with learning disabled children and adult stroke victims. Her book *Developing Cognitive and Creative Skills Through Art* was published in 1978.[17] She uses art as a means for strengthening conceptual, sequential, and spatial skills which are, in turn, the foundation of reading and mathematical skills. Silver asks rhetorically:

> Can handicapped children learn through art the concepts that are usually learned through talk? Can they express through drawings the thoughts and feelings they cannot put into words, and can their drawings provide useful clues to what they know and how they think or feel? Do they have as much aptitude for art as unimpaired children? Can educators use art to stimulate their cognitive or emotional growth without neglecting their creative growth? The answers to these questions may lie in special opportunities in art for educating children in general and handicapped children in particular. (Silver, 1978, p. 3)

Silver's work moves back and forth from theory (drawn from Jean Piaget, Jerome Bruner, and others who investigated cognition) to research and she provides case studies as well as statistical measures to make her points. She describes methods for testing for cognitive and creative skills as well as examples of art programs designed to accomplish her objectives. There are four such objectives that Silver identifies in working with any child or adult:

> Widening the range of communication, providing tasks that invite exploratory learning, providing tasks that are self-rewarding, and reinforcing emotional balance. These objectives seem appropriate both in art education and in

art therapy, regardless of whether the students are handicapped or normal, children or adults. (p. 108)

Silver's methods of assessment are considerably different from those of other writers discussed thus far. The Silver Drawing Test is built on the idea that "drawings can be used to assess the ability to solve conceptual problems" (Silver, 1990, p. 7). The Stimulus Drawings Test (1989b) presents a set of fifty line drawings to an individual who is told to "choose two drawings, imagine something happening between them, and show what is happening in a drawing of your own" (Silver, 1988, p. 8). The Draw-a-Story Test (1988) is used to screen for depression and emotional needs and uses 14 Stimulus Drawings from the other two instruments. Each test has its corresponding guidelines and rating scales for comparing the responses and submitting them to statistical analysis. The basic rationale for the Stimulus Drawings is that people "perceive the same stimulus drawings differently, that perceptions are influenced by personal experiences, and that response drawings reflect facets of personality in ways that can be quantified" (Silver, 1988, p. 8).

When asked to assess her contribution to the field, Silver wrote: "I feel it is probably in exploring ways to develop cognitive and creative skills nonverbally and to assess skills and attitudes that may escape detection through language" (Silver, 1985, p. 31).

Harriet Wadeson:
An Eclectic Approach

Harriet Wadeson met Hanna Yaxa Kwiatkowska and went to work with her in 1961 at the National Institute of Mental Health (NIMH) in Bethesda, Maryland, where Wadeson remained until 1975. However, she dates her actual entrance into the art therapy field as 1949:

> I first encountered art therapy in 1949 when I volunteered to work at St. Elizabeths Hospital in Washington, DC, during a college summer. The art teacher there, Prentiss Taylor, had been socked in the jaw by a criminal patient, so I took over his art groups. I didn't know art therapy could become a profession for me, so I remained an artist who wished to be a therapist. In 1961, several jobs, a marriage and two children later, I met Hanna Kwiatkowska. (Wadeson, 1985, p. 31)

Simultaneous with her work at NIMH, Wadeson attended classes at the Washington School of Psychiatry. Describing herself as having a "backwards training" by becoming an art therapist first and then a psychotherapist, Wadeson cites her patients as her most important source of learning:

> I believe my most significant teachers were the patients with whom I worked. I came to "know" through the accumulation of experience. Depression, for example was not merely aggression turned inward.... I understood the complexities of depression through my experience with over one hundred depressed patients with whom I had worked intimately, seeing their worlds in their pictures. (Wadeson, 1980, p. 30)

Wadeson's first publication "Communication Through Painting in a Therapy Group" appeared in the *Bulletin of Art Therapy* in 1964.[18] Her book *Art Psychotherapy* was published in 1980, *The Dynamics of Art Psychotherapy* in 1987, and *Advances in Art Therapy* (with Jean Durkin and Dorine Perach) in 1989. She is particularly known for her work with hospitalized patients and her innovative techniques for working with couples. Since 1970 she has been a teacher of art therapy and currently directs the Master's degree program in art therapy at the University of Illinois at Chicago.

Wadeson states that she uses an "eclectic approach" (Wadeson, 1987b). In her early years, she was most influenced by Freud. As she learned more and worked with patients, her theoretical basis became more influenced by phenomenology and the human potential movement. She also began to weave aspects of existentialism, Gestalt psychology, Jungian analytical psychology, and behaviorism as well as aspects of Erikson's developmental model and group therapy theory into her framework for art therapy. Wadeson writes:

> The power of an eclectic approach is the personal nature of its development. Nothing is taken for granted. It is not simply because I believe that many theories have something to offer, nor that any one theory may be too limiting—although I find both to be true—that I chose to be eclectic. (p. 299)

Wadeson continues:

> I believe theory to be an essential foundation to our work. An eclectic approach respects the contributions of many theorists and enables the clinician to draw on many sources of knowledge. It places a great deal of responsibility on the therapist to form a functional synthesis, integrating theories with one another and applying them to practice in the most efficacious way. (p. 312)

In *Art Psychotherapy*, Wadeson states that her approach is humanistic, existential, and phenomenological (Wadeson, 1980, p. xi). However, it is clear that she also uses aspects of other theories mentioned above.

Working as a primary therapist, she applies theories based on the clients' interpretation of their own work.

> I see psychotherapy as primarily an educational process to help people with problems in living rather than as a treatment for a disease. The educational process is not the traditional cognitive model, but rather an affectually oriented facilitation of emotional growth. (p. xi)

Wadeson stresses need for an art therapy theory that would integrate human psychology, creative art expression, and the meaning of visual imagery, but she does not begin to theorize. She does go so far as to say that:

> The client's creativity, as well as the therapist's, encompasses the entire art psychotherapeutic process. Such is the case in any form of therapy. In art therapy, however, the medium of expression is an art form, thereby encouraging a more focused creativity than otherwise. Since expression in visual imagery encourages production of fantasy material,...there is stimulation of some of the deeper layers of consciousness, bringing to bear on the creative processes richer resources than may be ordinarily available. (p. 7)

Wadeson's personal goal for each of her clients is to learn to accept and love themselves. Each client's goal, however, may be different. Goal setting is a cooperative effort between therapist and client.

> The point I wish to emphasize is that the art therapist sets goals based on the population and the conditions of the setting in which he or she works. The structure [of the therapy] then is established to enhance these goals. If a goal is dealing with a family crisis, then all family members may participate and be requested to draw pictures related to the crisis situation. If long-term insight-oriented psychotherapy is intended, then an individual may be seen alone on an ongoing basis using spontaneous picture-making. If socialization is an objective, then group projects or at least group sharing about individual art expressions may be encouraged, and so forth. (p. 17)

Wadeson does not interpret the picture for the client but encourages the client to discuss the image and to tutor her in its meaning. "The patients' verbal explanations and free associations provided abundant data so that interpretations and speculations have been minimal" (pp. 118–119). Although Wadeson does not interpret, she may facilitate the understanding of the images by asking open-ended questions. She tries to help clients to explore further by asking them to fantasize about their pictures.

It is the role of the art therapist to be accepting, non-judgmental, and understanding, and to provide a loving relationship. She is the empathic bridge between the images and the corrective emotional experience. She provides a model for creativity and a model for personal relationships. Wadeson summarizes the therapeutic relationship by saying:

> [it] is a creative alliance in which the therapist accompanies the client on a portion of her journey for the purpose of helping her to relinquish perceptual and behavioral attitudes that are causing her pain and to replace them with new ones that will increase her joy in living and promote feelings of self-acceptance, self-worth, and self-love.... The therapist is a follower rather than a guide, taking the lead from the client who points out the territory to be explored and the directions to be taken. (p. 38)

Words are important to the education and discovery process as the client discusses her work. There should be a balance between the role of talking and the role of the image. Because talking is a linear communication and making an image is a spatial communication, the picture often tells more at a glance than a lengthy monologue. "Obviously words may be used to elaborate and associate to the art expression, but the essential message is conveyed in image form" (p. 9).

According to Wadeson, the therapeutic process, growth, and communication (rather than aesthetic value) are important. She feels it is vital to be accepting and nonjudgmental of the art product as well as the client.

With respect to the role of creativity in art therapy she says:

> There are some who believe that the quality of the art product is indicative of the degree of sublimation achieved [such as Kramer]. Followers of this school...propose that it is the synthesizing effect of the creative force that produces art therapy's beneficial effect. I do not hold with this belief. Although I have worked with many people who achieved clarity and direction seemingly unconsciously and almost mysteriously through their art expression, I have worked with many others whose art expression was minimal or undeveloped, who achieved important insights and changes in themselves through reflecting on their images. In either case, there is creativity involved, but not necessarily only the narrow artistic sublimation Kramer suggests. (p. 6)

Shaun McNiff:
Art Therapist as Shaman

Shaun McNiff is a Professor at The Institute for the Arts and Human Development at Lesley College in Cambridge, Massachusetts. His books include *The Arts and Psychotherapy* (1981), *Educating the Creative Arts Therapist* (1986), *The Fundamentals of Art Therapy* (1988), and *Depth Psychology of Art* (1989).

McNiff began his art therapy work at Danvers State Hospital in Hawthorne, Massachusetts. McNiff remembers:

> The hospital hired me at age 23 just after I left law school.... My grandmother, Margaret Tyndall, had worked as a volunteer at the hospital, conducting weekly activity groups and organizing large summer parties for the patients in her garden in Peabody. I am sure this family connection to the hospital helped me to get that first job. The director of volunteers in my grandmother's days had been promoted to director of personnel and he worshipped her and therefore concluded that there should be something of value in me. It was...a perfect place to learn.... I often think that my grandmother, who died when I was in college, arranged it all since I never consciously planned to be an art therapist. (McNiff, 1985, p. 30)

McNiff continues:

> Shortly after [I] start[ed] at Danvers Dr. Rudolf Arnheim, who at the time was Professor of the Psychology of Art at Harvard, became interested in my work. He supervised my graduate studies and introduced me to his friend Margaret Naumburg. (p. 30)

In contrast to the other writers discussed so far, McNiff is the primary proponent of a broad expressive arts approach to education and therapy which includes poetry, drama, music, and dance therapies along with visual art.[19] McNiff defines his point of view by saying:

> I am an advocate for the primacy of the artistic identity of the therapist and opposed to narrow specialization.... I have complete faith in the ability of "art," in its most intelligent forms, both specific and global, to define the profession. (p. 30)

McNiff's theory involves a range of views and theories drawn from throughout history:

> Those that have been convinced that the unconscious forces rule their lives are believing again in *the will* and the life of the spirit inside of and between people.... The willful person has the power to focus, to concentrate and perceive selectively, Most importantly, however, this person can transform material existence. This is where the great power of the arts in psychotherapy lies. Throughout time, art has shown that it can change, renew, and revalue the existing order. If art cannot physically eliminate the struggles of our lives, it can give significance and new meaning and a sense of active participation in the life process. (McNiff, 1981, pp. v–vi, emphasis in the original)

Expressive art therapy becomes a healing ritual, a dramatization and visualization of conflict. Conflict within this context takes form in symbols, myths, and rituals. It is exorcised and healed through an emotional catharsis. "Art therapy is a manifestation of an old and often suppressed religious tradition based upon creativity, imagination and participation in the artistic process" (McNiff, 1989, p. 5).

Using a transpersonal and humanistic viewpoint, McNiff presents an integration of all the arts in psychotherapy, an amalgam which he calls "expressive arts therapy" (McNiff, 1981, p. vii). Rather than seeing the expressive therapies as emerging from 20th century psychology and psychiatry, McNiff takes a cross-cultural and anthropological perspective to postulate that the artist is the descendent of the shaman:

> The ancient predecessor of the expressive arts therapist can be found in every region of the world in the person anthropologists call the shaman. In many ways an early group therapist, the shaman's work is a response to communal needs. The shaman serves as the intermediary between people and "forces" that must be engaged in order to influence the course of community life. Shamanism is characterized by a belief in the power of human beings to participate in a direct and personal relationship with the supernatural dynamic of life. (p. 3)

By taking this longer look at healing McNiff concludes that:

modern psychotherapeutic practices are but a tiny dot within the universe of humankind's efforts to renew and heal the psyche. We have so completely accepted contemporary notions of time, space, life, and death that we have forgotten how these ideas were themselves constructed....

Today's psychological reality is but one of the myriad theoretical constructs that have been invented through history to justify and explain existence. If one is unhappy with life as it is perceived, it rarely occurs to that person that one's perception of life can be changed and reconstructed in a way that offers personal meaning. (pp. ix–x)

McNiff contends that: "Artists are generally more sensitive to our power to define and maintain concepts of reality.... Art's greatest power lies in its ability to create, change, and sustain value" (p. x).

Furthermore, he sees important parallels in the way relationships are viewed by those psychotherapists who reject psychological determinism and by artists:

Humanistic psychotherapy and art have in common a commitment to give order to changing experience by understanding the relationship of one dynamic occurrence to another. Their field of reference is open and all participants move in relation to each other. The illusion of the therapist as fixed to a constant position of observation is removed. With this unmasking the therapist's personal process and changing observations within the therapeutic moment are as vital as those of the client. (p. xii)

As for the specific value of the visual arts in therapy, McNiff states that they include:

> the introduction of visual communication in relationships...; spontaneous association to visual artworks...of feelings that are difficult to share verbally; the use of the *process* of creating art as a direct expression and catharsis...; the use of artworks as intermediary or "transitional" objects of communication...; the development of skills, personal competencies, and feelings of accomplishment...; and the encouragement of tangible development within a person's artistic expression as a means of furthering a more general integration of personality. (p. 155)

Interpretations of images are intuitive and changing because they are an image of life. Great caution must be taken not to abuse the image by applying a rigid, theory-bound interpretation. "The most significant interpretations are those that continue to act on us after the initial contact. They persist in their provocations of imagination while continuing to evoke the sensibility of the original image" (McNiff, 1989, p. 92).

The art therapist as inquirer, facilitator, and active explorer of art engages in a search for the individual and collective soul. The healer/therapist heals by "immersing the person and the group in the unity of the collective soul" (McNiff, 1981, p. 6). The therapist, as artist, must be a model of spontaneous and open expression. "The art therapist is an artist who attends to others, to images and to the soul. Attention to the self is an integral part of the discipline but it does not dominate the artist's social mission" (McNiff, 1989, p. 93).

Verbal and visual communication are integrated parts of all expressive modalities. Verbal responses often take the form of storytelling. Psychological language is avoided; its use is viewed as a defensive reaction:

> Talking can be both an avoidance of depth as well as a mode of deepening. Because we have done so much with talking in art therapy and psychotherapy as a whole, I am increasingly committed to researching the silent dialogue with art materials.... Talking takes the form of story telling within our training groups. (McNiff, 1986, p. 136)

The arts are important only as they express the flow of the person's feelings and not as technically finished products. They are "sacramental actions that symbolically represents the mysteries and intensities of inner experience" (McNiff, 1981, p. xxii).

Aina O. Nucho:

A Psychocybernetic View

Aina O. Nucho is a Professor at the University of Maryland School of Social Work and Community Planning where she teaches graduate-level courses in clinical methods with individuals, families, and groups. She holds a doctorate from Bryn Mawr College.

Nucho's art therapy is based in general systems theory. She uses Norbert Wiener's concept of "cybernetics" as the basis for her "psychocybernetic" model. Cybernetics is "the study of processes that make purposeful goal achievement of various systems possible. The principles of cybernetics permit the construction of goal-directed machines, robots, and computers" (Nucho, 1987, p. 17).

The way in which we are able to achieve this goal-direction is through a set of feedback loops. She describes two different types of feedback loops, negative and positive. Negative feedback prevents or decreases a certain activity while positive feedback encourages or increases the activity of the system. She cites cybernetics as the driving force in the development of biofeedback. Biofeedback aids patients in controlling and changing their physiological state which then changes the person's emotional and mental state. "The concept of cybernetics can be applied to all levels of organic and inorganic life. The very process of life is now understood as complex feedback loops" (p. 17).

In Nucho's model there are four phases to the therapeutic process: the Unfreezing phase, the Doing phase, the Dialoguing phase and the Ending phase. Within each phase, there is a specific set of goals to be achieved. In the Unfreezing phase the therapist focuses on giving the client information to make him/her feel more at ease with the art expression. This would include emphasizing the importance of the process rather than the aesthetic quality of the art and making sure that the client understands the amount of time allowed to create the drawing. The Doing phase is the actual creating; the Dialoguing phase is talking; and the Ending phase is closure.

> The psychocybernetic model of art therapy postulates that people are purposeful, information-seeking and information-processing behavioral systems. Art therapy, in light of psychocybernetics, may be thought of as an information processing enterprise. From this perspective, art therapy may be defined as the process of cultivating and explicating the internally produced signal system in the form of images that arise in response to the various experiences in life. (p. 20)

The goal in the psychocybernetic model is to aid clients in decoding their creations and finding a more appropriate way to assimilate and accommodate information.

Nucho describes two different approaches when examining the imagery contained in the client's work. They are the Ipsomatic versus Nomomatic Seeing. In the Nomomatic manner of seeing, the client's product is analyzed according to some theoretical approach. For instance, a therapist relying on a Freudian orientation would notice phallic shapes in the product, while a therapist using another approach might associate buttons in a self-portrait with dependency issues. Ipsomatic seeing is the core concept in the psychocybernetic model. This approach enables clients to decode their own creations.

> According to the psychocybernetic model, when working with the externalized imagery of clients, the task of the therapist is not to interpret the symbols contained in the imagery. Rather it is to facilitate the client's own seeing and understanding of those symbols. (p. 97)

Information constantly arrives from the different senses. The person has to sort out, codify, and integrate this new information with existing information in the system. When the information is not integrated, it becomes noise and not messages. Also, when there is an overload of information the system automatically makes it more manageable by condensing it into images.

> The job of the therapist is not to impart some specific philosophy of life. Rather it is to help the clients discern their own inner designs from their previous experiences in life and to understand their various obligations and aspirations. This thinking is compatible with the existential stream of ideas which views the development of the person as being molded by the commitments and future intentions rather than exclusively by past experiences. (p. 97)

Furthermore, Nucho states that "The task of the therapist is to assist the client in consolidating the information derived from various life experiences in order to construct internal frames of reference for appropriate pursuit of goal-directed behavior" (p. 20).

In addition, the therapist's role is to encourage the client to restore delight in primary forms of creativity.

> Therapy, it seems, is an activity that is akin to midwifery. The therapist assists in the process of delivery but the delivery is limited to that which the client has conceived and eventually will have to cherish and care for. (p. 97)

Nucho does not use the term transference in her writing. She does, however, speak of the relationship between the client and the therapist. And, "by paying attention to both channels of information processing in their clients and in themselves, therapists can work far more effectively than when only the verbal means of information exchange are heeded" (p. 95).

To Nucho talking is an important part of the therapeutic process. She underscores that it is a form of feedback to the system. In her framework a good therapist can facilitate the verbal discussion of the product even when the client seems to have nothing further to say. The therapist is able to introduce themes verbally that were only depicted by implication in the artwork. Nucho says that the Doing phase for children will be much longer than the Dialoguing phase. Conversely, in adults, the Dialoguing phase may be longer than the Doing phase.

> Even though the dialoguing process will not capture all the nuances contained in the visual creation, it still has value because it facilitates the process of codifying and integrating the new information with the information already stored in the system. (p. 172)

Rather than being concerned with an aesthetically pleasing product, Nucho's focus is on primary creativity. It is in the creative process that we can begin to understand how a person is hampered by information which emits conflicting messages.

> When applying the psychocybernetic model of intervention, we attempt to stimulate the primary creativity rather than the secondary type creativity. We ask clients to work spontaneously and fairly rapidly, without worrying about polishing and perfecting their creations. What matters is the process of stimulating imagination and what the client experiences during this phase of activity rather than what the finished product looks like. (p. 98)

Jungian Art Therapy Writers

The group of Jungian art therapists is relatively small in a field seemingly dominated by Freudian ideas. However, we speculate that Jung's influence has been fairly widespread although inconspicuous and not easily defined. It was mentioned earlier that Naumburg claimed no strict allegiance to Freud or Jung. But Jungian ideas seemed to take hold among art therapists in England more readily than in the United States. According to Edwards,

> Naumburg gives most space to Jung in *Schizophrenic Art* (1950) although this is mostly confined to a discussion of *Mythology of the Soul* by Baynes (1940), which includes two long art psychotherapy case histories. Baynes, who

had worked closely with Jung in the 1930s was a major influence, through Irene Champernowne, on the establishment of art therapy in Britain. (Edwards, 1987, p. 95)

Edwards also suggests that there is a strong emotional component influencing the selection of a theory to follow:

> Questions of loyalty figured strongly in the early days of psychoanalysis and tend to persist, not only in the literature, but also in the handling of knowledge and insight by successive generations of therapists. Since the quarrel between Freud and Jung was accompanied by such bitterness, it is not surprising that little attention should have been given to the insights of each school by the followers of the other. (p. 97)

Given the dominance of the Freudian model in the United States, it is no surprise that the Jungian art therapy literature is relatively limited compared with the psychoanalytically oriented literature. However, there are several articles, chapters, and books that provide a theoretical frame for Jungian art therapists.

One such book is Margaret Frings Keyes' *The Inward Journey: Art As Therapy for You* (1974). Throughout her work Keyes offers directives accompanied by vignettes which reveal how her clients were able to use them. She speaks of the indirect nature of the

Jungian approach and how these ideas unfold in art therapy:

> Art therapy does not answer the questions. It provides a process to clarify and deepen the questions, an awareness of how the individual here and now participates in creating his life conditions, and it points to some options that might be chosen. There are no highly visible models for this task. It is an individual journey. The individual has to take back parts of himself which he dislikes and does not want to see. He has to differentiate his own path from the ways of unthinking conformity to what is done by most people. (Keyes, 1974, p. 4)

As was pointed out in Chapter 1, Jung was highly interested in the mandala and several of the writers on Jungian art therapy at least mention the mandala in their writing. In her book Keyes includes a whole section on mandalas followed by ideas for directives. She relates that Jung described constructing a mandala as a self-healing process through which the psyche maintains its sanity and nurtures its own growth. "It stands for the deity as well as the self since it reflects the image of the godhead in the unfolded creation in nature and in man" (p. 58). Several authors (Brekke & Ireland, 1980; Slegelis, 1987) have written on the powerful use of the mandala in art therapy.

In addition to the *Inward Journey*, Keyes also wrote two articles, one on the shadow archetype (1976) and another on Dante and the tasks of individuation (1978). Several other authors (Benveniste, 1983; Musick, 1976; Nez, 1991; and Wittels, 1982) have also written on the use of archetypes in art therapy.

In Judith Rubin's *Approaches to Art Therapy* (1987a), two chapters were devoted to Jungian theory in art therapy. One chapter, written by Michael Edwards, entitled "Jungian Analytic Art Therapy," delves into the history of Jungian theory and how it is applied in art therapy.

> The symbolic image, for Jung, is its own best explanation; the unconscious does not lie, and it is only the ego which sometimes needs to defend itself against the truth. The image reveals its meaning when it is "accepted" as a projection which virtually speaks for itself, but in a way that is characteristic of its inherent nature. This acceptance of the unconscious image is not passive; it is treated neither as a symptom nor as a work of art. A relationship is encouraged between the image and its maker, by actively stimulating imaginative inquiry and dialogue, the essence of "active imagination." (Edwards, 1987, p. 98)

In addition, Edwards discusses Jungian archetypes and symbolism, and how the theory relates to art therapy practice.

In Jungian analytic therapy there is a tendency for certain archetypal themes to present themselves in an almost predictable sequence. How this happens will vary with every individual, but certainly quite often the early stages of therapy deal with the shadow, the denied and sometimes feared part of the personality that roughly corresponds, according to Jung, to the contents of the Freudian personal unconscious. (p. 105)

Edwards views Freud's major contribution to art therapy as the concept of latent content while Jung's was "to treat such images as communications from the psyche to be understood on their own terms and on many levels" (p. 112).

The other chapter was written by Edith Wallace, who was also one of the editors of *The Arts in Psychotherapy*, along with publishing several articles on Jungian art therapy (Wallace, 1975, 1980). Wallace describes a message from the depths of the unconscious as irrational, highly emotional, and "if we can be detached enough, it can become a dialogue between conscious and unconscious" (Wallace, 1987, p. 115). She outlines the process of facilitating this dialogue using art therapy:

The progression can then be from (1) emotionality to (2) a specific emotion, which may find expression in (3) an image, which can reduce the violence of the emotion; the image may be explained in (4) words, which represent articulation necessary for conscious understanding—a message received. (p. 115)

She writes of how Jung understood the consequences of not recognizing the images embedded in the unconscious.

In *Memories, Dreams, Reflections*, [Jung writes expressly: "The images of the unconscious place a great responsibility upon a man. Failure to understand them, or shirking of ethical responsibility, deprives him of his wholeness and imposes a painful fragmentariness on his life." (p. 117)

Jungian art therapy is a process to reestablish contact with a deeper self, from which emerges a feeling of wholeness. Partially due to the Jungian approach centering on the creative process in understanding the unconscious, many of Jung's ideas have been absorbed naturally into general art therapy theory without attribution.

Vija Bergs Lusebrink:
Imagery and Visual Expression

Imagery and Visual Expression in Therapy (1990) by Vija Bergs Lusebrink investigates a broad spectrum of theories and relates them to imagery and visual expression. In discussing the main influences in her work she states:

> The writings of art therapy pioneers [Naumburg, Ulman, and Rhyne] provided a framework for my own observations. Workshops and literature on guided imagery opened another door to the inner experience through images. The discovery of Jung's concept of archetypes helped me to integrate images into a mind/body frame bridging from the biological roots of the archetypal images to the spiritual aspects of our existence. The validity of my beliefs in imagery and its expression through visual means was reinforced and elaborated upon by additional exposure to...the use of visual expression of symbolism and symbolic realignment,...and imagery in therapy...as well as by my own clients and my observations of their visual expressions. (Lusebrink, 1990, p. vii)

In her doctoral studies she investigated the psychophysiological aspects of imagery. The wide range of material surveyed by Lusebrink illustrates how many important ideas have developed in art therapy and related fields since Naumburg wrote her first work.

Lusebrink "explores the different components and developmental, cognitive, and emotional aspects of imagery, visual expression, and the interaction of the two" (p. viii). She investigates the various approaches to symbolism including that of Freud and Jung and demonstrates how symbols function on many levels.

Lusebrink and her colleague Sandra Kagin (Kagin and Lusebrink, 1978) took the various components of imagery, symbols, and visual expression and developed the Expressive Therapies Continuum (ETC):

> This model consists of four levels organized in a developmental sequence of image formation and information processing. The first three levels reflect the developmental sequence and increasing abstraction in information processing in the following sequence: kinesthetic/sensory level (K/S), perceptual/affective level (P/A), and cognitive/symbolic level (C/Sy). The fourth level, the creative level (CR), can be present at any of the previous levels and may involve synthesis of all the other levels.... These same levels of organization can be applied to expression in other modalities, such as movement or expression through sound and rhythm. (Lusebrink, 1990, p. 92)

According to Lusebrink, "The interaction and transition between the different levels of the ETC can be described from a systems perspective" (p. 114). For each level there are certain "characteristics, healing dimensions, and emergent functions" (p. 119). Likewise, there are "manifestations of pathology" which show a "lack of interaction" between the levels of the ETC model (p.

122). Specific therapeutic strategies are suggested to counteract each of these disconnections.

In applying her systems perspective to the two poles of the art therapy field, Lusebrink says that:

> [in] *art as therapy*, the visual expressions through art media lead to self-regulation. The visual expressions... combine interaction on the different levels: The kinesthetic/sensory level is involved in the interaction with the media; the perceptual level provides the visual organization of stimuli into forms; the affect is amplified through the color and images used; the cognitive level of information processing deals with the organization of expression through sequencing of steps and problem solving; the symbolic level is manifested through the symbolic meaning of the images; and the final product of the expression attests to the presence of creative activity.
>
> In *art psychotherapy* the emphasis may be on a particular level as a starting point for the exploration of the disruption of functioning. The intrinsic qualities of the media influence differentially the levels of information processing involved and the portrayal of the images on different levels of expression. (pp. 242–243, emphasis in the original)

Notes:

[1] Harms wrote several early papers on the therapeutic use of art (Harms, 1944, 1947, 1948) and he stated that he "was one of the first who tried to standardize pictorial language for diagnostic purposes" (*Art Psychotherapy, 1*, 2, p. ii).

[2] Myra Levick gave a summary of the journal's history in 1986 (*The Arts in Psychotherapy, 13*, pp. 5–8). Harms had told her of his dream to start such a journal at a meeting of the American Society of the Expression of Psychopathology. Hahnemann Medical College was going to sponsor this journal but was unable to do so because of "administrative circumstances" (*Art Psychotherapy, 1*, 2, p. iii).

[3] The plan to have the American Art Therapy Association own the *American Journal of Art Therapy* collapsed in 1983. For details on the end of the affiliation see *AATA Newsletter, 13*, p. 2, April 1983.

[4] The first bibliography was produced under the auspices of the National Institute of Mental Health and the Alcohol, Drug Abuse and Mental Health Administra-

tion (ADAMHA) and was one of the first instances of recognition by the federal government of the field.

5 With their permission we have used portions of a paper written by Asawa, Bosky, Hass-Cohen, Kleiman, Roje, and Spector (1990) in the first-year art therapy literature class at Loyola Marymount University taught by Debra Linesch.

6 See Chapter 1 for Naumburg's background and education.

7 Pat Allen (1983) tells of Naumburg's "eclectic" interests in such areas as biofeedback and psychic research, and her knowledge of "world culture, art history, and of religion, especially Eastern religion." A list of Naumburg's publications follows Allen's article.

8 For more detailed discussions of different perspectives on the role of transference and countertransference in art therapy see Agell et al. (1981) and Levick (1983b). Considerable time at art therapy conferences and space in art therapy journals has been devoted to discussing this topic since the handling of transference

in *art psychotherapy* is different from that in the *art as therapy* approach.

[9] For more on Kramer's background see Chapter 2.

[10] For more on Ulman's background see Chapter 2.

[11] For more details about the specific art materials and the standardization of the Ulman Personality Assessment Procedure see Ulman, 1975d, pp. 362–364.

[12] For more on Kwiatkowska's background see Chapter 2.

[13] See Chapter 2 for those tasks.

[14] Landgarten's most recent book is on a multicultural assessment using magazine collage (1993).

[15] Janie Rhyne's book *The Gestalt Art Experience* was also published in 1973.

[16] For more on Rhyne's position regarding transference see Agell et al. (1981).

[17] In the third edition of this book (1989a) Silver adds an epilogue which provides a summary of research completed since the first edition.

18 This paper was published under the name Harriet Sinrod (1964).

19 See Agell and McNiff (1982) for a debate on whether art therapists should use only visual art or should combine it with dance, music, poetry, and/or drama.

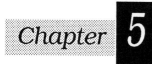
Building
on the Past

In preceding chapters we have attempted to provide an historical account of how the practice and profession of art therapy developed from 1935 to the present. Unquestionably, the most important event of the period was the formation of the American Art Therapy Association in 1969.

Many art therapists from those early days said that since they worked alone, they thought they had invented art therapy by themselves. Later, primarily through Elinor Ulman's journal, they were pleased to find others like themselves with whom they could form a professional community. Helen Landgarten remembers when she discovered that there were others like her:

One of the residents at the county hospital told me there was a *Bulletin of Art Therapy*. I back ordered all the issues. I had another friend doing a little art therapy and I thought we were the only ones in the world until I got the journal and found out there were people on the East Coast doing the same thing I was doing.... I've always been grateful to Elinor because of the journal. It was my lifeline.... Many of us thought we were the only ones.... I came to Louisville and met other real live art therapists and that was very important to me. (1975)

In discussing her experience of thinking "you're the only one," Landgarten said she believes such a feeling speaks to the strength and integral spirit of art therapy and of the centrality of art in the lives of those who have chosen to be in the field. She imagines that, even now, there are those in more isolated places who have never heard of the organized art therapy field but have found through their own experiences the usefulness of art in and as therapy and who are applying this knowledge to work with people (personal communication, 1986).

Despite some opposition to the formation of a national association, Myra Levick and Paul Fink hosted an organizational meeting in Philadelphia in December 1967. The American Art Therapy Association was established June 27, 1969, in Louisville, Kentucky, and Levick was elected its first President. In the next two decades, AATA established professional standards which provided a basis for the national registration of art therapists; developed guidelines for academic, clinical, and institute training programs; and instituted a procedure whereby those training programs meeting specific education guidelines could receive AATA's endorsement as "Approved" programs.[1] Originally organized around educational and clinical issues, AATA has increasingly moved into the political arena to fight for art therapists on matters such as state licensing, inclusion in civil service job classifications, and insurance coverage for art therapy services.

The American Art Therapy Association brought together a group of vociferous, artistic individualists with strong, and often contradictory, viewpoints. Many of the arguments voiced in the early conferences and journal articles, such as how to define the field, continue in some form or another to this day.

During the same time, there has been an explosion of educational programs for art therapists. The first Master's level art therapy program in the country seems to have been started by Dr. Roger White in 1957 at the University of Louisville. However, after about 1959, the program became inactive until 1969. Thus, Myra Levick would contend that the Master's program that began at Hahnemann Hospital in 1967 was the first (Levick,

1986, p. 187). Today, training programs reflect diverse theoretical viewpoints and often represent the strong convictions of the programs' founders, many of whom are still actively engaged in educating the next generations. Both Kramer's and Naumburg's methods remain strong components of the training programs. In addition, educators have begun giving attention to those types of skills necessary for art therapists to function as primary caregivers.

Art therapists have gained employment in an increasingly wide variety of settings, working with diverse populations, age groups, and problems. In addition to having jobs in psychiatric hospitals, art therapists are working in outpatient clinics, community mental health centers, residential treatment facilities, therapeutic and public schools, geriatric institutions, and private practice. By the mid-1980s, art therapy was used with families, sexually abused children, and the physically disabled. Some enterprising art therapists were beginning to explore art therapy applications in business settings.

With the expanding interest in art therapy and the burgeoning of training programs came a proliferation of art therapy literature which reflected considerable diversity in theoretical orientation and in case material. By 1985, there were three journals, and two comprehensive, annotated bibliographies had been published under the auspices of the National Institute of Mental Health.

The last decade was one of transition and challenge. There was a severe erosion of federal and state budgets for mental health programs during the Reagan and Bush administrations. The economy grew worse. Poverty and the underclass increased as did societal violence and depression. For the art therapist this now means increasingly difficult caseloads, clients with more profound psychopathology, crumbling resources, flagging clinical support, and, at times, morale difficulties. While art therapists continue to gain professional and public respect, the time of national expansiveness in mental health programs seen during the 1970s is over. Perhaps, the pioneering spirit embodied by the first art therapists will need come to the fore once again.

The *idea* of somehow combining *art* and *therapy* had existed for a long time in many individuals' minds. However, it was not until certain crucial factors such as deinstitutionalization, medications for psychosis, new therapy techniques, and the development of other mental health professions came together that a network could be developed in which the new profession formed.

Art therapy was created by people with strong personalities who used their creativity, energy, and personal resources to give shape, substance, and meaning to the new profession. They had courage, endurance, and, probably, some degree of naïveté because they did not know the problems they faced. Undauntingly, they often fought each other. They were born in a time in which American dreams of accomplishment and achievement were believed to provide a sufficient basis for ultimate success. The social struggles based on race, class, and gender which today threaten to shred the fabric of American life were mostly invisible then. From those fires of considerable creativity came the spirit of the survivor. To talk about these important women and men is to talk about the values and mores of those earlier times. The apparently freewheeling evolution of art therapy in the United States must be understood within the social context of a specific historical period, with particular motivating forces and constraints.

We will end this long trek through the past by placing the development of art therapy within the context of societal and cultural forces of the times. After that, our last task will be to attempt to give some shape and meaning to the 50-year process of transforming art therapy from something practiced by isolated individuals into an important, if still relatively unknown and small, profession. To do this, we will examine some of the economic, intellectual, and sociological factors from our past which have implications for our future.

The Great Depression & the Works Progress Administration

Art therapy was born into a climate in which, for the first time in this country, the arts and artists were involved with social and economic issues in an important way. This involvement in broader matters provided an important grounding for the new profession. While present-day arguments rage over the paucity of public support and government censorship of the arts, the idea that there should be federal and state subsidies of the arts seems such a given that we hardly remember how such programs began.

During the despair of the severe economic depression of the mid-1930s, one of the most remarkable social experiments of our national history came into being. On April 8, 1935, the Works Progress Administration (WPA), created by Henry Hopkins under Franklin D. Roosevelt's New Deal, was established. The WPA was, quite simply, a relief project through which money was given out in the form of salaries for work done by people using skills they already had. Less than one percent of the WPA budget was devoted to the arts but the WPA arts projects, which included the Federal Theater, Federal Music Project, Federal Art Project, and Federal Writers Project, employed 40,000 artists by the end of 1935.[2] The visionary Hopkins insisted that artists were as deserving of help as other indigent people. It was assumed that artists whose income was below the poverty level would be pleased to work for subsidy and that the American people would be happy to see the results of their labor if they were available at an affordable price. One congressman said, "The object of the WPA is to relieve distress and prevent suffering by providing work. The purpose is not the culture of the population." Yet, develop culture it did. For example, many playwrights, actors (such as Orson Wells), and technicians who became central to the American theater received their start and vital experience in the Federal Theater.

Some time before becoming an art therapist, Mary Huntoon returned in 1931 to Topeka, Kansas, after having spent 10 years as an artist in Europe. From 1934 to 1938, she was the Director of the Federal Art Project in Kansas.[3] It was in 1946 (after World War II) that Huntoon established the Department of Art, Physical Medicine, and Rehabilitation at Winter Veterans Hospital and began her research and writing in art therapy. We can speculate that Huntoon's experience and her background of the arts as integrally wedded to the necessities and realities of the social milieu had a deep impact on her and was carried with her into the work at Winter Hospital. Her own history as an early-day artist/social activist in the Federal Art Project thus provided Huntoon a model from which to develop her art therapy. This crucial, formative discovery and experience of social applications of the arts and their profound capacity for change is a prototypical story echoed by many art therapists through the years. It is often the motivation which leads people into the profession. We hear it repeated today by students in art therapy programs who proclaim, "I want to develop my art to help people."

Freud & Dewey:
Psychoanalysis & Progressive Education

The emergence and evolution of psychoanalysis as a dominant form of treatment in the United States in the beginning of the 20th century provided a fertile ground for developing a therapy which could offer a remarkable method for contacting the unconscious by providing images of that internal and often deeply hidden landscape. Freud's psychological investigations into his own psyche and those of his patients provided him with the material from which he created a dynamic psychology and a model for a theory of personality which has had the power to hold considerable sway in Western thought and to become one of the most important intellectual forces of the 20th century. In 1909, Freud was invited to speak at Clark University. His writings, translated by A. A. Brill, began to be published in the United States. The first translation of *The Interpretation of Dreams* appeared in 1913. Freud's conviction that the images and symbols of our dreams had meaning and were the disguised messages from the unconscious provided a powerful conceptual *raison d'être* for art therapy. Moreover, as interest in psychoanalysis spread in this country and its advocates in the intellectual community increased, more people, including artists, became convinced of its usefulness and intrigued with the products elicited through the method of free association.

Margaret Naumburg was born 26 years after Freud. One year after the publication of *The Interpretation of Dreams* in the United States, Naumburg founded the Walden School in New York, dedicated to a progressive educational philosophy based on psychoanalytic principles. Naumburg underwent analysis herself and many New York analysts including Brill sent their children to the school. Also, Naumburg was analyzed by Brill.

Through the efforts of Naumburg and others, progressive education, based largely on John Dewey's philosophy, became another important cornerstone for early art therapy practice. Dewey saw that the problems of education are connected to social, political, economic, and cultural problems. Thus, school becomes not so much a place where pupils go to simply acquire knowledge, as a place to carry on a way of life. It is an ideal community in which students practice cooperative interaction and self-government. A progressive school is viewed as a working model of democracy. Eschewing the Cartesian mind/body split and favoring an approach which emphasizes the total person, Dewey formulated an education based in meaningful experience and creative expression rather than on rigid intellectual methods (Dewey, 1958; Johnson, Dupuis, & Johansen, 1973). Progressive education is pragmatic, related to life, and process-oriented. It remains an important concept in the armamentarium of educational philosophies and most recently appeared prominently in the widespread educational reform movements of the late 1960s and 1970s which stressed the "whole child" in "the open classroom" and making education relevant to real life. Such ideas are obviously relevant to art therapy.

The Women's Movement as an Influence on Art Therapy

While there is no acknowledgment in the art therapy literature of the influence of the women's movement on the field, we believe that art therapy's evolution has shadowed this movement which has been centrally important in the 20th century. Art therapy has been created and developed largely by women and has suffered from many of the oppressive external and internalized constraints inherent in sexist conditions. And yet, art therapy's growth since the 1960s argues for its position as one of the most important new mental health professions to emerge since that time. It has a relevant predecessor in the social work profession with its commitment to solving social problems in the individual and in society. Social work is also a profession developed primarily by women.

When the question arises of why there are so few men in the field, the answer typically offered is that men do not tend to venture into low-paying professions with relatively low prestige. It is also suggested that the large numbers of women in the art therapy profession serve to keep away men who might enter it, in that they may perceive a "women's profession" as less powerful and important. Surely, there is some truth in those ideas, but we believe the reality to be more complex and more interesting. If women are the relational creatures that many writers and researchers would have us believe, it stands to reason that women quite naturally (and perhaps inherently) understand the connection of all that they do with the social and relational worlds around them and are driven to use their talents and skills in this way. Whether this is genetically or culturally determined, women use their talents for nurturing. It is not surprising, therefore, that women artists or women with an artistic bent would choose to use their skills in working with people.

The early art therapists had their own nurturers, mentors who, typically, were male psychiatrists fascinated with visual art and with the potential of imagery within therapeutic work. Mary Huntoon had Karl Menninger, Margaret Naumburg had Nolan D. C. Lewis, Myra Levick had Paul Fink, and Helen Landgarten had Saul Brown. The men "discovered" them, taught them, and helped them attain positions of importance and prominence. Also, it is not surprising, that in the male-dominated medical hierarchy of mental health, art therapists would have a long, hard struggle to establish standards of practice, education, and pay scales on a par with those of other mental health professionals. The struggle to be perceived as equal professional colleagues is certain to continue in a social and political climate in which the arts are often discounted and in which women and their nurturing roles are devalued.

With Paul Fink's help, Myra Levick provided the drive necessary to establish the American Art Therapy Association. As was described in preceding chapters, on-going arguments built on deep and passionate ideological convictions characterized the formation of the Association. But it should not be overlooked that, without a doubt, AATA gave the creative, energetic women who began it an arena in which to test themselves and to gain organizational skills and experience which would hold them in good stead as they developed educational and clinical programs across the country. At times, the depth of the internal struggles within AATA had the quality and intensity of a battle between good and evil. Junge (1992) notes the continuing ideological battle in the field between the proponents of *art as therapy* and *art psychotherapy* as emerging from an internalized dialectical model involving power and control. She speculates that the battles within AATA served to keep the participants locked in combat with each other. The art therapists who created the organization tested themselves and their ideas against each other and it made them strong. However,

A dialectical model is a decidedly male model. The descriptive terms used are individualistic, competitive, non-relational and are often about war. The two sides of the dialectic coin speak not about dialogue or conversation. They are about two lawyers with loud voices trying to shout each other down.... We still live in a patriarchal society and often wear patriarchal garb without even noticing it. Most art therapists are women. This, of course, does not preclude internalized sexism from the culture and unconscious attachment to habitual male ways of thinking and being on which much of our formal (and informal and tacit) education has been based. (Junge, 1992, pp. 9–10)

Regarding the broader nature of conflict and its ramifications, group psychotherapist, theoretician, and researcher Irving Yalom writes:

Although our immediate association with conflict is negative—destruction, bitterness, war, violence—a moment of reflection brings to mind positive associations: conflict brings drama, excitement, change, and development to human life and societies. (Yalom, 1985, p. 352)

While the founders of the American Art Therapy Association strenuously fought with each other, they also served one another as important sources of support and connection. And thus, another way in which the development of art therapy could be viewed as part of the evolution of women in this country is through the important role models who have emerged and who have mentored the new generations of art therapists who are predominantly women. Second-generation art therapists have often had the privilege of women mentors. In their roles as educational program developers, teachers, supervisors, and clinical colleagues, art therapists in all regions of the country have offered fledglings the support and encouragement necessary to grow. They have also provided a compelling model of competent, successful, and creative professionals seeking to develop themselves and to establish themselves and their profession.

Women in our society, even today, often remain invisible. But precisely because women are ignored and, frequently, are outsiders, they may be uniquely free to find their own voices. They are also intrinsically linked through their own experience of difference with other marginalized outsiders. And to a great extent, art therapists remain still the outsiders among other mental health professionals. This outsider position is shared with many artists as well. But for the woman art therapist, the evolution of the practice and profession of art therapy recounted in this history provides confirmation of the essential meaning of the struggle. As she sought to change herself, she changed the community around her.

As she demanded more respect for herself and her work, she gained more respect. As she established her work as a visible and visual force to be reckoned with, she could be threatening and threatened. She could also prevail over adversity. It has been said that the personal is political; there is no one for whom this must be more clearly in the forefront of her consciousness than the woman art therapist.

The Changing Mental Health Climate

In addition to these economic and societal influences, a central factor giving impetus to the new profession has been the changing national climate in mental health theories and treatments in the second half of the 20th century. With the notable exception of Margaret Naumburg who often functioned as a primary therapist, most early art therapists found work in psychiatric hospitals as part of a treatment team or as a special kind of art teacher with children. Freud's ideas, imported from Europe and associated with the past, took on a kind of American pragmatism in their transplanted new life in those psychotherapies which evolved after World War II. These new therapies, including group therapy, were developed to treat returning veterans. From this type of treatment more and varied forms of therapies sprang up. Carl

Rogers' client-centered approach stressed awareness of the here-and-now, not the understanding of antecedent causes, as was the goal of psychoanalytic psychotherapy. The expression of feelings was encouraged as a natural outgrowth of this approach. Rogers foreshadowed the development of humanistic psychotherapy and the emergence of the growth-oriented human potential movement of the 1960s. The 1950s saw the development of behavioristic forms of therapy based on theories derived from the experimental work of B. F. Skinner.

With the stunning development of the major tranquilizers in 1954, a whole new approach to understanding and treating psychiatric illness became possible. Patients who had spent years warehoused in institutions were suddenly rehabilitated as if by magic and were able to return to their home communities. In those communities, outpatient services were planned to provide humane and cost-effective forms of psychotherapy and treatment. The Federal Mental Health Act of 1963 established community centers and storefronts for outpatient services, most of which were short-term and crisis-oriented in nature. Often, funding was withdrawn from long-term treatment programs. Another type of therapy that developed and began to grow in the 1960s was based on systems theory. Family therapy was first discussed at a national meeting in 1957. The individual was no longer considered the only unit of treatment; the social context and interpersonal relationships gained increasing prominence and importance.

In the halcyon days of the new approach to mental illness when the patients were being released from the hospitals into the community, it seemed as if there were sufficient funds for these new programs. But, there were never enough relevant services. However, the air was filled with remarkable hopefulness and optimism that a new day had dawned. Staffing the centers created a ready and expanding job market for many newly trained therapists including art therapists. These developments gave the art therapists of the 1960s important clinical experience and the impetus to start the first academic training programs.

Training programs and art therapists increased in great number during the 1970s and 1980s. By 1992 there were 32 academic training programs nationwide and a number of well respected institute and hospital-based clinical programs as well. From the 50 art therapists who attended the organizational meeting in 1968, the membership of the American Art Therapy Association has grown to over 4200 in 1994.

Moving Toward the Future

In the previous pages we have looked back to examine the factors which came together to provide the bedrock on which art therapy was based. Now it is time to project ourselves toward the future. We ask the questions "What can be done?" and "What should be done?" in the troubled world our profession faces.

On March 18, 1993, Governor Bruce King of New Mexico signed the Counseling and Therapy Practice Act. In so doing, King put into effect the first state licensure law[4] in the United States that included art therapy as a named profession and set standards for its practice. That this important event could occur in such a different time and climate than did the expansive and innovative years of art therapy's remarkable early growth, indicates the claim to professional legitimacy which art therapy can now rightfully make. While this is unquestionably a milestone for the profession and for the New Mexico art therapists who worked long and hard to make it happen, passage of this law may also paradoxically and symbolically signal art therapy's most difficult professional challenges to come. In its short and colorful history, art therapy has managed fairly effectively to tread the dangerous line between regulation and definition from the outside and its own individualistic self-definitions.

How individual art therapists and the professional organization handle these dilemmas in the years to come will largely determine the field's future as a vital enterprise. While they did not, of course, use the terminology, the early art therapists had the foresight to forego the conception of a melting pot definition of their theory and practice in favor of the liveliness of diversity in which difference was understood as important. Although the wars within the profession over its definition often appeared to be a fight to the death, in hindsight it can be seen that they provided energy and life, perhaps even insured survival. We propose that organized art therapy did not perish from internal bickering because different points of view were at least tolerated from the very beginning. Early art therapists refused to be subsumed under one single, limiting definition while astutely observing the mental health terrain. Thus, there remain many definitions of art therapy and arguments among their proponents will continue. And it seems clear that in the future art therapists will need to take firm control of developing the means to validate their work.

Today in the United States, we are in an era of economic despair, in a country rife with problems emerging from our great democratic experiment. Job cutbacks, budget slashing in mental health programs, low morale of employees, and increasing violence in the lives of many Americans (and in what remains of mental health systems) portend the worst. Mental health treatment which focuses on biological determinism as the main cause of mental illness and tends to discount psychotherapy may well threaten art therapy's very survival. At a time of such economic and moral challenge, there is the tendency to rigidify and overstructure in the effort to ward off chaos and maintain some balance. This threat can come from outside or it can even come from within. In its history, organized art therapy has had to be ever mindful of its relationship to other mental health professions and outside accrediting bodies and commissions. As a "new kid on the block" it needed to find a way to be accepted and acceptable while still retaining its heart and spirit. This has never been easy. For example, there has been encouragement for many years for art therapists to establish professional credibility by conducting empirical research modelled after the behaviorism embraced by academic psychology. This has been done at the same time as we have discounted and underemphasized our identity as therapeutic artists and our more natural proclivities toward imaginative, interpretive work and research. On the other side of the coin, a few years ago, when educational programs in California found it necessary to relate art therapy to the vastly changing and more rigidly structured state licensing laws to stay viable in the job market, the cries within the profession were loud about how the California programs had abandoned their art, even though this was not the case.

The American Art Therapy Association is currently setting up a certification process which will include standardized testing. While we understand and support the spirit propelling these developments as a wish to enhance quality and promote art therapy's acceptability within a radically shifting health care climate, we urge great caution and a thoughtful, considerate approach. In the years to come, art therapists will need to be particularly nimble contortionists to both continue to be players in the mental health arena and yet also retain enough of the freedom which gives spirit and heart to the endeavor of art therapy. In a time when the walls seem to be closing in, art therapy also needs visionaries, along with the pragmatists and the politicians, to lead the way. And we speculate that although they may appear radically different from the pioneering visionaries of art therapy's history, they will hold dear, as did their forebears, the qualities of creativity, innovation, and a commitment to the bettering of the human condition in a time of profound difficulties.

True creative work requires opportunities for choices and inner freedom.

This chapter is written on the eve of radical reforms in our health care system. We cannot now see what the future will bring. But this we know: in our troubled times, there will be unforeseen-as-yet opportunities for positive growth, if we can maneuver the hazardous terrain with sensitivity, ingenuity, patience, and plain old grit.

Art therapists bring the gifts of imagery, symbol-making, and ritual. We help to construct meaning and to understand it because, projected through the art media, we see the hidden chambers of inner worlds. Making visible the invisible is the first step toward change. The art therapist is akin to a magician who pulls bouquets of multicolored flowers from a seemingly empty, dark, and even dangerous top hat. These flowers are symbols that offer dreams of nurturance, sustenance, and continuity in the face of despair and even death, of permanence in the face of whirlwinds, of transformation, and above all, of hope. The magic wand, created of art materials and wielded with sensitivity and intelligence, lights the client's journey. This wand, shaped by the art therapist, is put into clients' hands so that they may create for themselves the magical colors and shapes of meaning.

These flowers are symbols of the means to change and reform one's world.

Howard Gruber wrote:

> Creative work must be in some ways kindred to the world, if not the world as it is, then the world as it will or might be. It flows out of the world and it flows back into it. Thus the creative person, to carry out the responsibility to self, the responsibility for inner integrity , must also in some way be responsive to the world. (1989, pp. 280–281)

Art therapists may have a particularly advantageous perspective from which to foster societal change in order to make a more humane and just world. Historically, they have used their creativity well in the service of the profession. Thus far, art therapy has shown itself to have the staying power of a piece of clay successfully fired in the kiln of history. For the future, as we have noted above, it will take considerable vigilance to not allow the spirit and flexibility of the exciting mix of art and therapy to be obliterated by outside forces. The problems ahead are not the easy ones. As Gruber says: "But how do we know what can be done? Only by pushing to the very limits of what is possible." (1989, p. 281)

Notes:

[1] The term *approved* is used when an organization verifies that an educational program meets specific requirements. The term *accredited* is used in higher education when an *accrediting body* gives its stamp.

[2] Some information for this section was culled from O'Conner and Brown (1978).

[3] Typical of WPA arts projects were murals on social themes in federal buildings such as courthouses and post offices.

[4] There are a few other state licensing laws which permit art therapists to qualify for licensing under other professional titles.

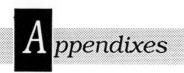
Appendixes

Chronology
Minutes of First Meeting
AATA Constitution
Job Description

Chronology

MAJOR EVENTS

1882   **Margaret Naumburg** is born in New York City.

1913   **Freud's** *The Interpretation of Dreams* is published in the United States.

1914   **Margaret Naumburg** founds the **Children's School** which becomes the **Walden School** in 1915. It is a progressive school established on psychoanalytic principles.

1920   **Florence Cane**, Naumburg's sister, comes to teach art at Walden. Naumburg leaves the directorship of the school.

1922   **Hans Prinzhorn's** book *Bildnerei Der Geisteskranken* (Artistry of the Mentally Ill) is published.

1925   **Nolan D. C. Lewis**, Director of the New York State Psychiatric Institute, uses free paintings with his adult patients.

The Rorschach Test, first published in Europe in 1921, is brought to the United States.

1926 **Florence Goodenough** designs the "Draw-A-Man" test, an intelligence test for children.

1928 **Naumburg** publishes her first book, *The Child and the World,* based on her experiences at the Walden School.

Late **Mary Huntoon** works under Karl Menninger at
1930s at the Veteran's Administration Hospital in Topeka, Kansas. Calls herself an art therapist and names what she does "dynamically oriented art therapy." (By this term she means paying attention to the psychodynamics of the case.)

Edith Kramer conducts art classes in Prague for children who are refugees from Nazi Germany. She sees the value of art in alleviating stress and trauma.

1938 **Naumburg** visits the Menninger Clinic to give a presentation. She meets with Mary Huntoon.

1940 **Naumburg** defines dynamically oriented art therapy as a method of releasing the unconscious by means of spontaneous art expression.

1939 **Edith Kramer** teaches art at the Little Red School
-41 in New York City, a private, progressive school.

1941 **Naumburg** meets **Nolan D. C. Lewis** and initiates a research program at the New York Psychiatric State Institute using dynamically oriented art therapy, first with behavior problem children and then with patients with schizophrenia. Her research lasts until 1946.

1942 **Don Jones**, a conscientious objector, works at Marlboro State Hospital in New Jersey. He collects patients' artwork and notices that art seems to hold great meaning for them. He remains there until 1946. He writes a book of patient art titled *PRN*.

1947 **Naumburg's** first art therapy book is published—*Studies of the "Free" Expression of Behavior Problem Children as a Means of Diagnosis and Therapy*.

The pioneering art educator Viktor Lowenfeld publishes what will become a classic about children's art, *Creative and Mental Growth*.

The *House-Tree-Person Test* is designed by **John Buck**.

1949 Psychologist **Karen Machover's** *Personality Projection in the Drawing of the Human Figure* is published.

1950 **Naumburg** publishes *Schizophrenic Art: Its Meaning in Psychotherapy*.

Don Jones teaches art classes in Kansas. Some of his students are psychiatrists and social workers from the Menninger Clinic; through them he meets Dr. Karl Menninger.

Edith Kramer begins teaching art at the Wiltwyck Home for Boys, a residential treatment center for emotionally disturbed boys in New York City.

Felice Cohen begins doing art therapy at the Houston State Psychiatric Hospital through her friend **Dr. Irving Kraft** who had read Naumburg and suggests that Cohen try art therapy.

1950s **Naumburg** gives training seminars in "The Techniques and Methods of Art Therapy" in New York, Philadelphia, Washington, and Cambridge, MA, to medical students, psychiatric hospital staff members, and other professionals. **Elinor Ulman** arranges the lectures in Washington, DC. **Hanna Yaxa Kwiatkowska** attends.

Elinor Ulman takes a position at the District of Columbia General Hospital in Washington, DC. She meets **Bernard I. Levy**, the Chief Psychologist.

1951 **Florence Cane's** book *The Artist in Each of Us* Is published.

Jones begins work as an art therapist at the Menninger Clinic. He remains there until 1966.

1952 **Florence Cane** dies.

1953 **Naumburg's** *Psychoneurotic Art Its Function in Psychotherapy* is published.

1954 **Dr. René Spitz**, an outstanding Freudian analyst, speaks as the principal discussant at a symposium on art therapy at the meetings of the American Orthopsychiatric Association.

1955 **Hanna Yaxa Kwiatkowska**, a Polish artist and sculptor, begins work at St. Elizabeths Hospital in Washington, DC.

1957 **Ulman** teaches "Introduction to Art Therapy" to psychiatrists, nurses, and social workers at the Washington School of Psychiatry.

Dr. Roger White initiates a Master's degree program in art therapy at the University of Louisville in the Departments of Art and Psychology. After graduating two students in 1959, the program becomes inactive for ten years.

1958 **Kramer's** first book *Art Therapy in a Children's Community* is published. Based on her work at Wiltwyck School it gives a second theoretical position for art therapy by focusing on the therapeutic properties of the creative process.

Two chapters by **Naumburg** are included in Emanuel Hammer's *The Clinical Application of Projective Drawings.*

Kwiatkowska joins the National Institute of Mental Health. She remains there for 14 years and develops innovative techniques in family art therapy.

The magazine *Scientific American* devotes a whole issue to the subject of creativity.

1959 "A Schizophrenic Patient's Response in Art Therapy to Changes in the Life of the Psychotherapist,"

Kwiatkowska's first paper (written with S. Perlin), is published.

1960   Robert Ault joins Don Jones at the Menninger Clinic.

A course in "Psychiatric Art Therapy" is given in the Department of Psychiatry at Temple University's School of Medicine by two psychiatrists, Roy Stern and Harold Winn.

1961   Elinor Ulman edits and publishes the *Bulletin of Art Therapy*, the first, and for twelve years the only, journal in the field. Isolated art therapists across the country discover the journal and consider it a lifeline.

Insania Pingens, a study of psychotic art, is published.

Harriet Wadeson comes to work with and be trained by Hanna Yaxa Kwiatkowska at the National Institute of Mental Health. In Kansas, Don Jones and Robert Ault dream of starting a national organization for art therapists.

1963   Ulman undertakes a survey of art therapists and finds only thirty-five in the United States and Canada.

1964   Kramer initiates a program in therapeutic art at the Jewish Guild for the Blind in New York.

Janie Rhyne goes back to school where she discovers Gestalt psychology and begins to integrate it with art.

1964 -65 With a $80,000 grant from the National Institute of Mental Health **Tarmo Pasto** in Sacramento, California, conducts a research study categorizing graphic imagery from institutionalized mental patients, prison inmates, and juvenile delinquents.

1966 Art therapists **Marge Howard, Elinor Ulman, Sandra Kagin,** and **Tarmo Pasto** attending the meetings of the International Society of Psychopathology of Expression in Washington, DC, talk of forming their own organization.

Naumburg's *Dynamically Oriented Art Therapy* is published.

1967 **Myra Levick** becomes Director of Adjunctive Therapies and Coordinator of the first graduate training program at Hahnemann Hospital and Medical College in Philadelphia.

A group of art therapists exhibit artwork of psychiatric patients at the American Psychiatric Association conference in Boston. The group includes **Naumburg, Kramer, Kwiatkowska, Jane Gilbert, Lynn Flexner Berger, Miryam Dergalis, Carolyn Refsnes Kniazzeh**, and **Myra Levick.** Levick's colleague **Paul Fink** from Hahnemann hosts the group for lunch. All agree that a national organization needs to be formed to define art therapy as a profession.

Don Jones leaves the Menninger Clinic to go to Harding Hospital in Ohio.

Helen Landgarten begins work as an art therapist on an adolescent unit at the Los Angeles County General Hospital. One year later, she becomes an art therapist at Mt. Sinai Hospital (which later becomes Thalians Community Mental Health Center, Cedars Sinai Hospital).

Myra Levick and **Paul Fink** host a series of lectures for art therapists at Hahnemann. About 50 attend. Despite some opposition, an *ad hoc* committee is formed to draw up a constitution and bylaws for a national organization of art therapists. Members of the committee are **Elinor Ulman, Myra Levick, Don Jones, Robert Ault,** and **Felice Cohen.**

1969 The American Art Therapy Association is voted into existence June 27, 1969, at a meeting in Louisville, Kentucky. Elected to the first Executive Board are **Myra Levick,** President; **Robert Ault,** President-Elect; **Marge Howard,** Treasurer; **Felice Cohen,** Secretary; **Elsie Muller,** Constitution Chair; **Helen Landgarten,** Public Information Chair; **Sandra Kagin,** Education Chair; **Don Jones,** Publications Chair; **Hanna Yaxa Kwiatkowska,** Research Chair; and **Ben Ploger,** Standards Chair. The first Honorary Life Membership is awarded to **Margaret Naumburg.** AATA is chartered in Oklahoma. Dues are $15.00. A newsletter is published.

1970 **AATA** holds its first annual conference at Airlie House, Warrenton, Virginia. **Margaret Naumburg** receives the Honorary Life Membership and makes a warm acceptance speech. The members decide to certify art therapists and plan a registration process.

The same day AATA is formed **Sandra Kagin** is hired to reactivate the art therapy program at the University of Louisville which had originally opened in 1957 and closed in 1959.

The *Bulletin of Art Therapy* changes its name to the *American Journal of Art Therapy.*

The first humanistically oriented art therapy program is started at the Pratt Institute, a free-standing art school in New York City. **Josef Garai** becomes the Director.

1971 **Edith Kramer's** second book, *Art Therapy with Children,* is published.

AATA's second conference is held in Milwaukee, Wisconsin.

Dr. Bernard Levy and **Elinor Ulman** begin the Master's program in art therapy at the George Washington University.

1973 **Guidelines for Education and Training** in art therapy are adopted by AATA.

A second journal, *The Arts in Psychotherapy,* edited by **Ernest Harms**, is begun.

Janie Rhyne's book *The Gestalt Art Experience* is published. It reflects an integration of Gestalt psychology and art therapy.

Self-Discovery Through Self-Expression, written by **Mala Betensky**, is published. It presents art therapy within a humanistic, phenomenological framework.

For the first time at the **Menninger Clinic**, art therapy is listed as a separate psychotherapeutic service. Previously, it was an activity therapy.

1973 The art therapy program at the University of Louisville headed by Sandra Kagin becomes the **Institute for Expressive Therapies** and includes all the arts.

1974 **Helen Landgarten** starts the first art therapy program on the West Coast at Immaculate Heart College in Los Angeles. Calling the program "Clinical Art Therapy," she trains art therapists to function as primary clinicians.

The *American Journal of Art Therapy* affiliates with AATA.

1975 Art therapy educators meet as a group for the first time, hosted by the George Washington University. This group will become the **International Convocation of Art Therapy Educators**.

Through its Education and Training Board AATA begins to endorse programs meeting its *Guidelines* as "Approved."

1977   There are now twenty-one art therapy training programs in the country.

1978   **Hanna Yaxa Kwiatkowska's** *Family Therapy and Evaluation Through Art* is published.

1979   **Kramer's** *Childhood and Art Therapy* is published.

1980   **Landgarten's** program moves to Loyola Marymount in Los Angeles.

        Hanna Yaxa Kwiatkowska dies.

        Harriet Wadeson's *Art Psychotherapy* is published.

1981   **Helen Landgarten's** *Clinical Art Therapy A Comprehensive Guide* and **Shaun McNiff's** *The Arts in Psychotherapy* are published.

1983   **Margaret Naumburg**, age 93, dies in her sleep in Boston.

        After a bitter battle, the *American Journal of Art Therapy* does not renew its affiliation with AATA. It will be published by Norwich University in Vermont. AATA publishes the first edition of its new journal *Art Therapy*. **Gary Barlow** is selected to serve as editor; **Linda Gantt** and **Mildred**

Lachman-Chapin had served as interim editors for the first issue.

1984 AATA is 15 years old.

1985 The list of educational offerings published by AATA includes 14 "Approved" programs, 24 universities and colleges offering art therapy programs and courses, eight graduate level certificate programs, five clinical programs, five institute programs, and 32 universities and colleges offering undergraduate art therapy degree programs with art therapy prerequisites.

1985 New generations of art therapists are finding employment in an increasingly wide variety of settings and are working with diverse age groups and problems.

1991 AATA joins the American Dance Therapy Association in urging passage of amendments to the Older Americans Act which name art, dance, and music therapy

1992 The United States Senate Special Committee on Aging holds a hearing on art and dance/movement therapy with older Americans.

The Older Americans Act (Public Law 102–375) is passed. For the first time art therapy is name specifically in federal legislation. Money appropriated for demonstration grants and res studies.

AATA membership reaches 4018. The number of "Approved" training programs is now 24.

AATA publishes its first monograph, *A Guide to Conducting Art Therapy Research.*

1993   AATA officially designates the Master's degree as the entry level for the profession.

New Mexico becomes the first state to offer licensure to art therapists under the Counselors and Therapists Practice Act. This is the first time art therapists have been named on their own (not under another profession's title) in a state licensing law.

1994   The American Art Therapy Association is 25 years old.

PRINCIPAL WRITERS

(Below are the titles and dates of the first publications on art therapy by these important writers along with their first published books. Complete information on these can be found in the References section, beginning on page 315.)

1942 **Don Jones**
-45 *PRN in a Mental Hospital Community* (paintings by his patients and by Jones) (Civilian Public Service Unit, 1945)

1947 **Margaret Naumburg**
Studies of the "Free" Art Expression of Behavior Problem Children and Adolescents as a Means of Diagnosis and Therapy (a collection of papers which had been published previously, beginning in 1943)

1949 **Mary Huntoon**
"The creative arts as therapy"

1958 **Edith Kramer**
Art Therapy in a Children's Community

1959 **Hanna Yaxa Kwiatkowska**
"A schizophrenic patient's response in art therapy to changes in the life of the psychotherapist"

1978 *Family Therapy and Evaluation Through Art*

1961 **Elinor Ulman**
Edits and publishes the *Bulletin of Art Therapy*

1964 **Harriet Wadeson** (as H. Sinrod)
"Communication through paintings in a therapy group"

1980 *Art Psychotherapy*

1967 **Myra Levick**
"The goals of the art therapist as compared to those of the art teacher"

1983 *They Could Not Talk & So They Drew*

1973 **Mala Betensky**
Self-Discovery Through Self-Expression

1973 **Janie Rhyne**
The Gestalt Art Experience

1973 **Judith Rubin**
"A diagnostic art interview"

1978 *Child Art Therapy*

1973 **Arthur Robbins**
"A psychoanalytical perspective towards the interrelationship of the creative process and the functions of an art therapist"

1976 *Creative Art Therapy* (with L. B. Sibley)

1974 **Margaret Keyes**
The Inward Journey Art as Psychotherapy for You

1975 **Helen Landgarten**
"Group art therapy for mothers and their daughters"

1981 *Clinical Art Therapy: A Comprehensive Guide*

1975 **Shaun McNiff**
"Video art therapy"

1981 *The arts and psychotherapy*

1975 **Edith Wallace**
"Creativity and Jungian thought"

1978   Rawley Silver
Developing Cognitive & Creative Sklls Through Art

1979   Aina Nucho
"Self-portraits and selected indicies of psychopathology of a group of heroin-addicted patients"

1989 *The Psychocybernetic Model of Art Therapy*

1990   Vija Bergs Lusebrink
Imagery & Visual Expression in Therapy

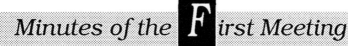

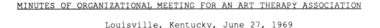

MINUTES OF ORGANIZATIONAL MEETING FOR AN ART THERAPY ASSOCIATION

Louisville, Kentucky, June 27, 1969

The meeting was called to order in the University of Louisville at 11:15 a.m. by Myra Levick, Chairman of the Ad Hoc Steering Committee of art therapists. Dean Warren Jones welcomed the group of about fifty art therapists, educators, psychologists, and psychiatrists on behalf of the University. Mrs. Levick next introduced Roger K. White, Assistant Professor of Psychiatry in the University of Louisville's School of Medicine, who has taken an interest in the organization of art therapists ever since the idea was broached in May,1968. Doctor White expressed his continuing support. Mrs. Levick then introduced the remaining members of the Ad Hoc Steering Committee: Robert Ault, Felice Cohen, Don Jones, and Elinor Ulman. A representative sample of letters received by committee members from people unable to attend the meeting but interested in its outcome was read by Elinor Ulman, Don Jones, and Felice Cohen.

Some recent developments influenced by the prospect of an art therapy organization were reported. They included the founding of local art therapy associations; favorable action on an art therapy research grant; interest on the part of universities in offering art therapy courses; the production of papers on art therapy by graduate students and professionals; increases in the number of applicants for already existing training courses; and a panel discussion on art therapy which was the first session on this subject ever held at an annual meeting of the American Psychiatric Association.

Robert Ault reported that $240.00 had been received in donations toward the Steering Committee's work since its formation in December, 1968. Expenditures of $49.00 consisted of $22.000 for a projector used at the American Psychiatric Association art therapy panel, and $27.00 paid the Menninger Foundation for printing and mailing, leaving on hand a balance of $191.00.

The Constitution and Bylaws unanimously recommended by the Ad Hoc Steering Committee were then laid before the meeting for discussion. They were introduced by the following Statement of Principle, read by Felice Cohen: "At the meeting of the duly elected Ad Hoc Steering Committee of the National Organization of Art Therapists it was resolved as a unanimous recommendation of the committee that: (1) A national organization for art therapists be formed on June 27, 1969, (2) and that the enclosed statement of Principle and Bylaws serve as the official documents of the Organization to be known as the American Art Therapy Association."

The Constitution was read by Mr. Jones and the Bylaws by Mr. Ault, as you have received under separate cover.

Mr. Ault moved and Mr. Jones seconded the motion that the Constitution and Bylaws be adopted as read.

The meeting adjourned for lunch at 12:30 p.m.
The afternoon session convened at 1:15 p.m.

Discussion of the Constitution and Bylaws touched on numerous questions of definition definitions of membership requirements, of functions and media included under the ter art therapy, and so on. Committee members pointed out that their aim had been to produce documents which would allow for the greatest possible openness and flexibilit so that movement toward stricter definition could proceed gradually on the basis of r adequate information about present practices, and in the light of future developments in the field. Potential members were urged to communicate with the Chairman of the Constitutional Committee at any time about modifications in the Constitution and Byla that may be desirable.

ome questions concerning job openings for graduates of present and contemplated training programs produced assurances that opportunities for trained art therapists re available and can be expected to increase.

The motion to adopt the proposed Constitution and Bylaws was passed by a unanimous vote Mrs. Cohen moved and Bernard I. Levy seconded the motion that nominations for officers and committee chairmen be made, the vote recorded, and the final election left open unt ballots could be distributed by mail and returns from absentees eligible to attend the meeting could be counted. After discussion, the motion was defeated in favor of electing officers and committee chairmen to take office immediately.

Before the floor was opened to nominations, Myra Levick announced the Ad Hoc Steering Committee's recommendation to the incoming Executive Committee that Margaret Naumburg be invited to become the Association's first Honorary Life Member. The announcement was greeted with applause, and approval of the recommendation was agreed upon by all present at the meeting..

Elections took place as follows:
President: Nominees were Myra Levick, Robert Ault, and Don Jones. Myra Levick was elected.
President Elect: Nominees were Robert Ault, Elsie Muller, Sandra Kagin, and Don Jones. Robert Ault was elected.
Secretary: Nominees were Felice Cohen and Elinor Ulman. Miss Ulman declined the nomination, and Mrs, Cohen was unanimously elected.
Treasurer: Margaret Howard and Don Jones were nominated. Mr. Jones declined the nomination and Mrs. Howard was unanimously elected.
Committee Chairmen:

Constitution: Don Jones and Elsie Muller were nominated; Mr. Jones withdrew in favor of Mrs. Muller, who was unanimously elected.

Finance: Paul J. Fink and Ben J. Ploger were nominated but both declined the nomination. Mrs. Roberta Capers, who was not present at the meeting, was unanimously elected. Should she refuse to serve, the Executive Committee will select a replacement

Membership: Bernard Stone was elected unanimously.

Publications: Don Jones was elected unanimously. Miss Ulman expressed interest in serving on this committee.

Education: Ben Ploger and Sandra Kagin were nominated; Sandra Kagin was elected Edith Kramer was suggested as an appropriate member of this committee because of her outstanding knowledge in the area of training for work in art therapy with children.

Public Information: Helen Landgarten and Elinor Ulman were nominated; Miss Ulman declined the nomination and Mrs. Landgarten was unanimously elected.

Research: Kay Pellock and Hanna Yaxa Kwiatkowska were nominated. Mrs. Pellock withdrew in favor of Mrs. Kwiatkowska, who was unanimously elected although not present at the meeting. In the event of her being unwilling to serve, the Executive Committee will select a replacement. Harriet Wadeson was mentioned as well qualified for this position. Kay Pellock and Mary Lee Alford expressed interest in serving on this committee.

Professional Standards: Kay Pellock and Ben Ploger nominated; Ben Ploger elec

It was mentioned that all who are interested in serving on a particular committee should communicate their wishes to the appropriate chairman.

It was suggested that the Membership Committee make efforts to recruit members from Canada.

A brief discussion indicated that those present favored the fall of the year rather than the summer as a date for future annual meetings.

It was announced that the Executive Committee will disseminate information to the organizational mailing list and will develop and announce plans for the Association's first Annual Meeting.

Those eligible for membership were invited to send dues to Mrs. Margaret Howard, Children's Medical Center, Tulsa, Oklahoma.

The meeting was adjourned at 3:45 p.m.

Elinor Ulman,
Secretary pro tem.

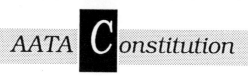

AATA *C*onstitution

CONSTITUTION

OF

THE AMERICAN ART THERAPY ASSOCIATION

JUNE, 1969

ARTICLE I

NAME

The name of the organization shall be the American Art Therapy Association.

ARTICLE II

Purpose and Objectives

Section I   The purpose of the Association shall include: (A) The progressive development of the use of art therapeutically, (B) The advancement of research interests, and standards of clinical practice, (C) To further the cause of developing criteria for training future therapists in diagnostic and therapeutic techniques, (D) Provide an appropriate vehicle through which an exchange of information and experiences might be shared by colleagues, (E) To coordinate the use of art therapeutically in private practice or institutional settings.

Section II   The Objectives of the Association shall be those which: (A) Aim treatment most effectively toward human welfare, improvement and rehabilitation, (B) The promoting of art therapy through all possible means, (C) Encouraging the development of professional standards for persons engaged in art therapy, (D) To conduct meetings, seminars and clinics to improve the effectiveness of those engaged in art therapy, (E) To encourage the development of professional training opportunities in art therapy, (F) To attract the interest and initiative of individuals to the field of art therapy.

ARTICLE III

MEMBERSHIPS

Section I   The memberships shall consist of such persons who shall make written application to become members and who shall pay membership dues. There shall be eight classes of individual memberships which include Active, Associate, Student, Contributing, Sustaining, Life, Patron, and Honorary Life.

Section II   Membership may also be applied for by regional State, Municipal, school, or other local organizations. The local organization may associate itself with the American Art Therapy Association free of dues, although individual members within the organization shall abide by the same membership criteria as outlined in Section I.

Section III   Membership privileges and annual dues shall be prescribed in the Bylaws of the Association.

ARTICLE IV

OFFICERS

Section I   The officers of the American Art Therapy Association shall be elected from the active membership. The authority and duty of each official shall be such as defined in the Bylaws.

Section II   The elective officers of the Association shall be a President, President-elect, a secretary, a treasurer, and an executive committee consisting of standing committee chairmen. They shall be elected by ballot during a regular annual meeting, and shall serve in office as described in the Bylaws.

Section III   No elective officer shall hold the same office for more than two terms.

Section IV   Elections shall be conducted as stated in the Bylaws.

Section V   The president, with consent of the majority of the officers and the executive committee shall make appointments as necessary, for terms also agreed upon by the Executive Committee.

ARTICLE V

STANDING COMMITTEES

Section I   Standing Committees shall consist of the following: Constitution, Finance, Membership, Publications, Education, Professional Standards, Public Information, and Research.

Section II   The organization and duties of the committee are outlined in the Bylaws.

ARTICLE VI

MEETINGS

Section I   Annual meetings of the Association shall be held at such a time and place as shall be determined by the officers and executive committees.

Section II   Notification of such annual meetings to be sent to the membership a minimum of sixty days prior to the designated day.

Section III   Special meetings of the officers and executive committee may be called at the request of a majority of those members and must state the specific business to be transacted.

ARTICLE VIII

QUORUM

Section I   A quorum shall consist of a majority of the officers, the Executive Committee, and those of the active membership present, the proposed amendments having been submitted to the membership at least four weeks in advance of the meeting.

ARTICLE VIII

AMENDMENTS

Section I   This constitution may be amended at any annual meeting by a two-thirds vote of the active membership, who may either be present or have submitted their vote by mail, the proposed amendments having been submitted to the membership at least four weeks in advance of the meeting.

Section II   Bylaws may be adopted, amended, or repealed at any session of an annual meeting by a two-thirds vote of the active membership who may either be present or have submitted their vote by mail, the proposed change having been submitted to the membership at least four weeks in advance of the meeting.

ARTICLE IX

DISSOLUTION OF ORGANIZATION

Section I   Should, for any reason, the Association be dissolved, any funds and properties belonging to the Association shall be returned to the constituents in proportion to the constituents' dues and contributions made to the Association in the current year.

ART THERAPIST:
Model Job Description

Definition

The art therapist treats individuals, couples, families, and groups through therapeutic art tasks. While the art therapy process utilizes art making as a means of nonverbal communication and expression, the art therapist will typically make use of verbal explorations and interventions as well. The art therapist may act as a primary therapist or as adjunctive within the treatment team, depending upon the needs of the institution and treatment objectives of the patient. He/she provides a range of services, including preventive services, diagnostic evaluation, assessment, and treatment using art therapy techniques, and process.

Application

The art therapist treats a variety of populations in diverse settings, including, but not limited to, the emotionally disturbed, the physically disabled, the elderly, the developmentally delayed, prisoners, and the drug dependent. Art therapists are employed in mental health facilities, both inpatient and outpatient, community mental health centers, family service agencies, rehabilitation centers, medical hospitals, corrections institutions, developmental centers, educational institutions, private practice, and other facilities.

Duties

Art therapists assist their clients in alleviating distress, reducing physical, emotional, behavioral, and social impairment, and promoting positive development. Within agency guidelines and professional standards, art therapists may provide any, or all, of the following: diagnostic evaluation; development of patient treatment plans, goals, and objectives; case management services; and therapeutic treatment. Art therapists also maintain appropriate charting, records, and periodic reports on patient progress as required by the agency, participate in professional staff meetings and conferences, and provide information and consultation regarding the client's clinical progress in the art therapy setting. Art therapists may also function as supervisors, administrators, consultants, and as expert witnesses.

Educational Requirements
(Training & Experience)
The American Art Therapy Association defines entry level into the profession at the Master's degree level. The art therapist will have graduated from a a two-year Master's degree program, or the equivalent, which will have included a minimum of 600 hours of supervised practicum experience. Some programs require 1000 hours of practicum. Those Master's, Institute, or Clinical programs which are approved by the American Art Therapy Association meet educational standards set forth by the Association. AATA also certifies the competency of individual art therapists who can meet the specific requirements of the Association. Art therapists certified by AATA are designated A. T. R. (Art Therapist, Registered).

> May 5, 1987
> Maxine Junge, MSW, LCSW, A.T.R.
> Chair, Clinical Committee

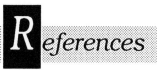eferences

Adamson, E. (1984). *Art as healing*. York Beach, ME: Nicolas-Hays.

Agell, G., Levick, M., Rhyne, J., Robbins, A., Rubin, J. A., Ulman, E., Wang, C., & Wilson, L. (1981). Transference and countertransference in art therapy. *American Journal of Art Therapy, 21,* 3–24.

Agell, G., & McNiff, S. (1982). Great debate: The place of art in art therapy. *American Journal of Art Therapy, 21,* 121–123.

Allen, P. (1983). The legacy of Margaret Naumburg. *Art Therapy: Journal of the American Art Therapy Association, 1,* 5–6.

American Art Therapy Association Pamphlet (1977). Mundelein, IL: American Art Therapy Association.

Anastasi, A., & Foley, J. (1940). A survey of the literature on artistic behavior in the abnormal: III. Spontaneous productions. *Psychological Monographs, 52,* 1–71.

Anastasi, A., & Foley, J. (1941a). A survey of the literature on artistic behavior in the abnormal: I. Historical and theoretical background. *Journal of General Psychology, 25,* 111–142.

Anastasi, A., & Foley, J. (1941b). A survey of the literature on artistic behavior in the abnormal: IV. Experimental investigations. *Journal of General Psychology, 23,* 187–237.

Arnheim, R. (1984). For Margaret Naumburg. *The Arts in Psychotherapy, 11,* 3–5.

Asawa, P., Bosky, J., Hass-Cohen, N., Kleiman, R., Roje, J., & Spector, R. (1990). Out on a limb. Unpublished paper. Los Angeles, CA: Loyola Marymount University.

Ault, R. (1970). Unpublished letter to Elinor Ulman, December 8. Topeka, KS: Archives of the American Art Therapy Association, Menninger Foundation Library.

Ault, R. (1975). An oral history: Art therapy pioneers [audio tape]. Louisville, KY: Department of History, University of Louisville.

Ault, R. (1977). Are you an artist or therapist—A professional dilemma of art therapists. In R. Shoemaker & S. Gonick-Barris (Eds.), *Creativity and the Art Therapist's Identity,* Proceedings of the 7th Annual AATA Conference. Baltimore, MD: American Art Therapy Association.

Ault, R. (1985). Personal communication with author.

Barlow, G. (1985). Personal communication with author.

Baynes, H. G. (1940). *The mythology of the soul: A research into the unconscious from schizophrenic dreams and drawings.* London: Williams & Wilkins.

Benveniste, P. (1983). The archetypal image of the mouth and its relation to autism. *The Arts in Psychotherapy, 10*, 99–112.

Betensky, M. (1971). Impressions of art therapy in Britain: A diary. *American Journal of Art Therapy, 10,* 75–86.

Betensky, M. (1973). *Self-discovery through self-expression: Use of art in psychotherapy with children and adolescents.* Springfield, IL: Charles C Thomas.

Betensky, M. (1987). Phenomenology of therapeutic art expression and art therapy. In J. A. Rubin (Ed.), *Approaches to art therapy.* New York, NY: John Wiley.

Brekke, J. & Ireland, M. S. (1980). The mandala in group psychotherapy, personal identity, and intimacy. *The Arts in Psychotherapy, 7,* 217–231.

Buck, J. (1948). The house, tree, person technique: A quantitative and qualitative scoring manual. *Clinical Psychology Monograph, 5,* 1–20.

Cane, F. (1929). Art and the child's essential nature. *Creative Art, 4,* (2), 120–126.

Cane, F. (1951/1983). *The artist in each of us*. Craftsbury Common, VT: Art Therapy Publications. [Originally published by Pantheon, New York, NY.]

Civilian Public Service Unit No. 63, (1945). *PRN in a mental hospital community*. Marlboro, NJ: Author.

Cocteau, J., Schmidt, G., Steck, H., & Bader, A. (1961). *Insania pingens [If this be madness]*. Basel: Ciba.

Cohen, F. (1970a). Unpublished letter to American Art Therapy Association Executive Board, December 3. Topeka, KS: Archives of the American Art Therapy Association, Menninger Foundation Library.

Cohen, F. (1970b). Letter. *American Art Therapy Association Newsletter, 1,* (4), 2.

Cohen, F. (1975a). An oral history: Art therapy pioneers. [audio tape]. Louisville, KY: Department of History, University of Louisville.

Cohen, F. (1975b). Introducing art therapy into a school system: Some problems. *Art Psychotherapy, 2,* 121–135.

Cohen, F. (1976). Art psychotherapy: The treatment of choice for a six-year-old boy with a transsexual syndrome. *Art Psychotherapy, 3,* 55–67.

Cohen, F., & Phelps, R. (1985). Incest markers in children's art work. *The Arts in Psychotherapy, 12,* 265–283.

Corsini, R. (Ed.). (1981). Handbook of innovative psychotherapies. New York, NY: John Wiley & Sons.

Day, J., & Kwiatkowska, H. Y. (1962). The psychiatric patient and his "well" sibling: A comparison though their art productions. *Bulletin of Art Therapy, 2,* 51–66.

Dax, E. C. (1953). *Experimental studies in psychiatric art.* London: Faber.

Detre, K. C., Frank, T., Kniazzeh, C. R., Robinson, M. C., Rubin, J. A., & Ulman, E. (1983). Roots of art therapy: Margaret Naumburg (1890–1983) and Florence Cane (1882–1952)—A family portrait. *American Journal of Art Therapy, 22,* 111–123.

Dewey, J. (1958). *Art as experience.* London: Putnam.

Drachnik, C. (1992). Unpublished letter to the author, June 5.

Edwards, M. (1987). Jungian analytic art therapy. In J. A. Rubin (Ed.). *Approaches to art therapy.* New York, NY: Brunner/Mazel.

Elkisch, P. (1948). The scribbling game—a projective method. *The Nervous Child, 7,* 247.

Fink, P., Goldman, M. J., & Levick, M. F. (1967). Art therapy, a new discipline. *Pennsylvania Medicine, 70,* 60–66.

Freud, S. (1963). Dreams. In J. Strachey (Ed. and trans.). *New introductory lectures on psychoanalysis.* (Vol. XV, Part II). London: Hogarth Press.

Friedman, L. J. (1990). *Menninger: The family and the clinic.* New York, NY: Alfred A. Knopf.

Gantt, L. (1991). Personal communication with the author.

Gantt, L., & Schmal, M.(1974). *Art therapy: A bibliography,* January 1940–June 1973, Rockville, MD: National Institute of Mental Health, DHEW Publication No.(ADM) 74–51.

Garai, J. E. (1971). The humanistic approach to art therapy and creativity and development. Paper presented at the 2nd annual conference of the American Art Therapy Association, Milwaukee, WI.

Garai, J. (1985). Meet the ole timers: Perspectives on the American Art Therapy Association. Messages in Art. Program of the 16th Annual Conference for the American Art Therapy Association, New Orleans, LA.

Geller, S. (1980). The unique dynamics of an art therapist and her client. Unpublished paper, April.

Goodenough, F. (1926). *Measurement of intelligence by drawings*. New York, NY: Harcourt, Brace, & World.

Groth-Marnat, G. (1990). *Handbook of psychological assessment* (2nd ed.). New York, NY: Wiley-Interscience.

Gruber, H. (1989). Creativity and human survival. In D. Wallace & H. Gruber (Eds.), *Creative people at work*. New York, NY: Oxford University Press.

Hagaman S. (1986). Mary Huntoon: Pioneering art therapist. *American Journal of Art Therapy, 24,* 92–96.

Hammer, E. (Ed.) (1958). *The clinical application of projective drawings*. Springfield, IL: Charles C Thomas.

Harms, E. (1944). The arts as applied psychotherapy. *Occupt. & Rehab., 23,* 51–61.

Harms, E. (1947). Child art as an aid in the diagnosis of juvenile neuroses. *American Journal of Orthopsychiatry, 11,* 191–210.

Harms, E. (1948). Awakening into consciousness of subconscious collective symbolism as a therapeutic procedure. *Journal of Child Psychiatry, 1,* 208–238.

Harris, D. (1963). *Children's drawings as measures of intellectual maturity*. New York, NY: Harcourt, Brace, & World.

Hill, A. (1948). *Art versus illness: A story of art therapy*. London: Allen & Unwin.

Hill, A. (1951). *Painting out illness*. London: Williams & Norgate.

Holden, W. M. (1965). Ars Gratia Hominis: The world of Tarmo Pasto. *California Mental Health Progress*, 5–9.

Huntoon Archives (n.d.). Kansas collection of Spencer Library. Lawrence, KS: University of Kansas.

Huntoon, M. (1948). Creative art therapy showing clinical classifications of art used as treatment. Unpublished manuscript. Lawrence, KS: University of Kansas, Huntoon Archives.

Huntoon, M. (1949). The creative arts as therapy. *Bulletin of the Menninger Clinic, 13,* 198–203.

Huntoon, M. (1953). Art therapy for patients in the acute section of Winter VA hospital. *VA Department of Medicine & Surgery Information Bulletin, 10,* 29–33.

Huntoon, M. (1959). Art for therapy's sake. *Mental Hospital,* January, 20.

Introducing... (1961). *Bulletin of Art Therapy, 1,* 2, 5–6.

Jakab, I. (Ed.). (1968). *Psychiatry and art.* Proceedings of the IVth International Colloquium of Psychopathology of Expression, Washington, DC, 1966. New York, NY & Basel: S. Karger.

Jakab, I. (Ed.). (1969). *Art interpretation and art therapy.* Proceedings of the Vth International Colloquium of Psychopathology of Expression, Los Angeles, California. New York, NY & Basel: S. Karger.

Jakab, I. (Ed.). (1971). *Psychiatry and art,* Vol. 3. Proceedings of the 4th annual meeting of the American Society of Psychopathology of Expression. New York, NY & Basel: S. Karger.

Johnson, J., Dupuis, H., & Johansen, V. (1973). *Introduction to the foundations of American education.* Boston, MA: Allyn & Bacon.

Jones, D. (1947). *Tunnel.* Unpublished manuscript.

Jones, D. (1962). Art and the troubled mind. *Menninger Quarterly, 16,* 12–19.

Jones, D. (1970, November–December). Editor's notes. *American Art Therapy Association Newsletter, 1*(4).

Jones, D. (1975). An oral history: Art therapy pioneers [audio tape]. Louisville, KY: Department of History, University of Louisville.

Jones, D. (1983). An art therapist's personal record. *Art Therapy: Journal of the American Art Therapy Association, 1,* 22–25.

Jones, D. (1993). Personal communication (telephone call with L. Gantt, September 9).

Jordan, H. (1988). An interview with Elinor Ulman. *American Journal of Art Therapy, 26,* 107–112.

Jung, C. (1916). *Psychology of the unconscious* (B. Hinkle, transl.). London. [Published in 1956 as *Symbols of transformation,* in the *Collected works,* vol. 5, Bollingen Series XX. Princeton, NJ: Princeton University.]

Jung, C. (1954). *The aims of psychotherapy. The practice of psychotherapy,* Bollingen Series XX. New York, NY: Pantheon.

Jung, C. (1972). *Mandala symbolism.* Princeton, NJ: Princeton University Press.

Junge, M. (1987). Research notes on Mary Huntoon from Huntoon collection, Lawrence, KS: University of Kansas.

Junge, M. (1992). Reconsidering the wars between art and therapy and reconceptualizing a model for our profession. Unpublished paper.

Kagin, S., & Lusebrink, V. (1978). The Expressive Therapies Continuum. *Art Psychotherapy, 5,* 171–179.

Keyes, M. F. (1974). *The inward journey: Art as psychotherapy for you.* Millbrae, CA: Celestial Arts Press. [Published in 1983 in a revised edition with the title *Inward journey: Art as therapy.* LaSalle, IL: Open Court Publishing.]

Keyes, M. F. (1976). Art processes evoking awareness of the shadow archetype. *Art Psychotherapy, 3,* 77–80.

Keyes, M. F. (1978). Dante and the tasks of individuation. *Art Psychotherapy, 5,* 17–22.

Kiell, N. (1965). *Psychiatry and psychology in the visual arts and aesthetics: A bibliography.* Madison, WI: University of Wisconsin Press.

Kramer, E. (1958). *Art therapy in a children's community.* New York, NY: Charles C Thomas.

Kramer, E. (1961). Art and emptiness: New problems in art education and art therapy. *Bulletin of Art Therapy, 1,* 7–16.

Kramer, E. (1962). Art education and emptiness. *Bulletin of Art Therapy, 1,* 20–24.

Kramer, E. (1963). The problem of quality in art. *Bulletin of Art Therapy, 3,* 3–19.

Kramer, E. (1964). A critique of Kurt Eissler's *Leonardo da Vinci*. *Bulletin of Art Therapy, 4,* 20–33.

Kramer, E. (1965). Art therapy and the severely disturbed gifted child. *Bulletin of Art Therapy, 5,* 3–20.

Kramer, E. (1966). Art and craft. *Bulletin of Art Therapy, 5,* 149–152.

Kramer, E. (1967). The problem of quality in art. II: Stereotypes. *Bulletin of Art Therapy, 6,* 151–171.

Kramer, E. (1968). Autobiography of a ten-year-old: Introduction and comment. *Bulletin of Art Therapy, 7,* 119–130.

Kramer, E. (1970). Letter. *American Art Therapy Association Newsletter, 1,* (4).

Kramer, E. (1971a). Unpublished letter to Felice Cohen, February 25. Topeka, KS: Archives of the American Art Therapy Association, Menninger Foundation Library.

Kramer, E. (1971b). *Art as therapy with children.* New York, NY: Schocken.

Kramer, E. (1972). The practice of art therapy with children. *American Journal of Art Therapy, 11,* 89–110.

Kramer, E. (1979). *Childhood and art therapy.* New York, NY: Schocken.

Kramer, E. (1986). The art therapist's third hand: Reflections on art, art therapy, and society at large. *American Journal of Art Therapy, 24,* 71–86.

Kramer, E., (1990). Personal communication with J. Roje.

Kramer, E. (1992a). Tributes. *American Journal of Art Therapy, 30,* 67.

Kramer, E. (1992b). Reflections on the evolution of human perception: Implications for the understanding of the visual arts and of the visual products of art therapy. *American Journal of Art Therapy, 30,* 126–142.

Kramer, E., & Scher, J. (1983). An art therapy evaluation session for children. *American Journal of Art Therapy, 23,* 3–12.

Kramer, E., & Ulman, E. (1976). Editorial—Art therapy: Further explorations and definitions. *American Journal of Art Therapy, 16,* 2 & 42.

Kramer, E., & Ulman, E. (1977). Postscript to Halsey's "Freud on the nature of art." *American Journal of Art Therapy, 17,* 21–22.

Kwiatkowska, H. Y. (1962). Family art therapy: Experiments with a new technique. *Bulletin of Art Therapy, 1,* 3–15.

Kwiatkowska, H. Y. (1967). The use of families' art productions for psychiatric evaluation. *Bulletin of Art Therapy, 6,* 52–69.

Kwiatkowska, H. Y. (1978). *Family therapy and evaluation through art.* Springfield, IL: Charles C Thomas.

Kwiatkowska, H. Y., Day, J., & Wynne, L. C. (1962). The schizophrenic patient, his parents, and siblings: Observations through family art therapy. Catalogue of exhibit presented at the annual meeting of the American Psychiatric Association. Washington, DC: U.S. Department of Health, Education, & Welfare, Public Health Service.

Kwiatkowska, H. Y., & Perlin, S. (1959). A schizophrenic patient's response in art therapy to changes in the life of the psychotherapist. DHEW Publication No. NIH-33807. Bethesda, MD: U. S. Public Health Service.

Landgarten, H. (1975a). An oral history: Art therapy pioneers [audio tape]. Louisville, KY: Department of History, University of Louisville.

Landgarten, H. (1975b). Group art therapy for mothers and their daughters. *American Journal of Art Therapy, 14,* 2.

Landgarten, H. (1981). *Clinical art therapy: A comprehensive guide.* New York, NY: Brunner/Mazel.

Landgarten, H. (1986). Personal communication with author.

Landgarten, H. (1987). *Family art psychotherapy: A clinical guide and casebook.* New York, NY: Brunner/Mazel.

Landgarten, H. (1993). *Magazine photo collage: A multicultural assessment and treatment technique.* New York, NY: Brunner/Mazel.

Landgarten, H., & Lubbers, D. (Eds.). (1991). *Adult art psychotherapy: Issues and applications.* New York, NY: Brunner/Mazel.

Levick, M. F. (1967). The goals of the art therapist as compared to those of the art teacher. *Journal of Albert Einstein Medical Center, 15,* 157–170.

Levick, M. F. (1970a). Unpublished letter to Elinor Ulman, December 3. Topeka, KS: Archives of the American Art Therapy Association, Menninger Foundation Library.

Levick, M. F. (1970b). President's message. *American Art Therapy Association Newsletter, 1,* (4).

Levick, M. F. (1971a). Letter in the reader's forum. *American Journal of Art Therapy, 10,* 74, 98–99.

Levick, M. F. (1971b). Unpublished letter to Edith Kramer, November 9. Topeka, KS: Archives of the American Art Therapy Association, Menninger Foundation Library.

Levick, M. F. (1973). Introduction to art therapy. *Philadelphia Medicine, 69* (7).

Levick, M. F. (1975a). An oral history: Art therapy pioneers [audio tape]. Louisville, KY: Department of History, University of Louisville.

Levick, M. F. (1975b). Transference and countertransference as manifested in graphic productions. *Art Psychotherapy, 2,* 203–215.

Levick, M. F. (1975c). Art in psychotherapy. In J. Masserman (Ed.), *Current psychiatric therapies,* (Vol. 15, pp. 93–99). New York, NY: Grune & Stratton.

Levick, M. F. (1981). Art therapy: An overview. In R. Corsini (Ed.), *Handbook of innovative psychotherapies.* New York, NY: John Wiley.

Levick, M. F. (1983a). *They could not talk and so they drew: Children's styles of coping and thinking.* Springfield, IL: Charles C Thomas.

Levick, M. (Ed.), (1983b). Transference and countertransference in the fine art of therapy. In L. Gantt & S. Whitman (Eds.), *The fine art of therapy.* Proceedings of the 11th Annual Conference of the American

Art Therapy Association. Alexandria, VA: American Art Therapy Association.

Levick, M. F. (1985). Meet the ole timers: Perspectives on the American Art Therapy Association. Messages in Art. Program of the 16th Annual Conference for the American Art Therapy Association, New Orleans, LA.

Levick, M. F. (1986). *Mommy, Daddy, look what I'm saying: What children are telling you through their art* (with D. Wheeler). New York, NY: M. Evans.

Levick, M. F., Goldman, M., & Fink, P. (1967). Training for art therapists: Community mental health center and college of art join forces. *Bulletin of Art Therapy, 6,* 121–124.

Lewis, N. D. C. (1925). The practical value of graphic art in personality studies. I. An introductory presentation of the possibilities. *Psychoanalytic Review, 12,* 316–322.

Lewis, N. D. C. (1928). Graphic art productions in schizophrenia. *Pro. A. Res. Nervous & Mental Diseases, 5,* 344–368.

Lowenfeld, V. (1964). *Creative and mental growth* (5th ed.). New York, NY: MacMillan.

Lusebrink, V. B. (1990). *Imagery and visual expression in therapy.* New York, NY: Plenum Press.

Lyle, J., & Shaw, R. F. (1937). Encouraging fantasy expression in children. *Bulletin of the Menninger Clinic, 1,* 78–86.

MacGregor, J. (1983). Paul-Max Simon: The father of art and psychiatry. *Art Therapy: Journal of the American Art Therapy Association, 1,* 8–20.

MacGregor, J. (1989). *The discovery of the art of the insane.* Lawrenceville, NJ: Princeton University.

Machover, K. (1949). *Personality projection in the drawing of the human figure.* Springfield, IL: Charles C Thomas.

Mahler, M., Pine, F., & Bergman, A. (1975). *The psychological birth of the human infant.* New York, NY: Basic.

Malchiodi, C. (1990). *Breaking the silence: Art therapy with children from violent homes.* New York, NY: Brunner/Mazel.

McMahan, J. (1989). An interview with Edith Kramer. *American Journal of Art Therapy, 27,* 107–114.

McNiff, S. (1975). Video art therapy. *Art Psychotherapy, 2,* 55–63.

McNiff, S. (1979). The art therapist as artist. In L. Gantt, G. Forrest, D. Silverman, & R. Shoemaker (Eds.), *Art therapy: Expanding horizons.* Proceedings of the 9th Annual AATA Conference. Baltimore, MD: American Art Therapy Association.

McNiff, S. (1981). *The arts and psychotherapy.* Springfield, IL: Charles C Thomas.

McNiff, S. (1985). Meet the ole timers: Perspectives on the American Art Therapy Association. Messages in Art. Program of the 16th Annual Conference for the American Art Therapy Association, New Orleans, LA.

McNiff, S. (1986). *Educating the creative arts therapist: A profile of the profession.* Springfield, IL: Charles C Thomas.

McNiff, S. (1988). *Fundamentals of art therapy.* Springfield, IL: Charles C Thomas.

McNiff, S. (1989). *Depth psychology of art.* Springfield, IL: Charles C Thomas.

Meares, A. (1957). *Hypnography: A study in the therapeutic use of hypnotic painting.* Springfield, IL: Charles C Thomas.

Meares, A. (1958). *The door of serenity.* Springfield, IL: Charles C Thomas.

Meares, A. (1960). *Shapes of sanity: A study in the therapeutic use of modelling in waking and hypnotic states.* Springfield, IL: Charles C Thomas.

Moore, R. (1981). *Art therapy in mental health* (Literature survey series, no. 3). DHHS Publication No. (ADM) 81-1162. Rockville, MD: National Institute of Mental Health.

Muller, E. (1968). Family group art therapy: Treatment of choice for a specific case. In I. Jakab (Ed.), *Psychiatry and art*. Proceedings of the IVth International Colloquium of Psychopathology of Expression, Washington, DC, 1966. New York, NY & Basel: S. Karger.

Musick, P. (1976). Primitive percepts and collective creativity. *Art Psychotherapy, 3*, 43–50.

Naumburg, M. (1928). *The child and the world*. New York, NY: Harcourt Brace.

Naumburg, M. (1943). Children's art expression and war. *The Nervous Child, 2,* 360–373.

Naumburg, M. (1944). The drawings of an adolescent girl suffering from conversion hysteria with amnesia. *Psychiatric Quarterly, 18,* 197–224.

Naumburg, M. (1944). A study of the art expression of a behavior problem boy as an aid in diagnosis and therapy. *The Nervous Child, 3,* 277–319.

Naumburg, M. (1945a). A study of the psychodynamics of the art work of a nine-year-old behavior problem boy. *Journal of Nervous and Mental Disease, 101,* 28–64.

Naumburg, M. (1945b). Phantasy and reality in the art expression of behavior problem children. In N. D. C. Lewis & B. L. Pacella (Eds.), *Modern trends in child psychiatry.* New York, NY: International Universities Press.

Naumburg, M. (1946). A study of the art work of a behavior problem boy as it relates to ego development and sexual enlightenment. *Psychiatric Quarterly, 20,* 74–112.

Naumburg, M. (1947). Studies of the "free" art expression of behavior problem children and adolescents as a means of diagnosis and therapy. *Nervous and Mental Disease Monographs,* No. 71. New York, NY: Coolidge Foundation. [Revised edition printed in 1973; see Naumburg, 1973.]

Naumburg, M. (1950). *Schizophrenic art: Its meaning in psychotherapy.* New York, NY: Grune & Stratton.

Naumburg, M. (1953). *Psychoneurotic art: Its function in psychotherapy.* New York, NY: Grune & Stratton.

Naumburg, M. (1958a). Art therapy: Its scope and function. In E. F. Hammer (Ed.), *The clinical application of projective drawings.* Springfield, IL: Charles C Thomas.

Naumburg, M. (1958b). Art therapy with a seventeen-year-old schizophrenic girl. In E. F. Hammer (Ed.), *The clinical application of projective drawings*. Springfield, IL: Charles C Thomas.

Naumburg, M. (1966). *Dynamically oriented art therapy: Its principles and practice*. New York, NY: Grune & Stratton. [Reprinted in 1987. Chicago, IL: Magnolia Street.]

Naumburg, M. (1973). *An introduction to art therapy: Studies of the "free" art expression of behavior problem children and adolescents as a means of diagnosis and therapy*. New York, NY & London: Teachers College Press, Columbia University.

News... (1965). A Fulbright travel award (for Hanna Yaxa Kwiatkowska). *Bulletin of Art Therapy, 4* , 74–76.

Nez, D. (1991). Persephone's return: Archetypal art therapy and the treatment of a survivor of abuse. *The Arts in Psychotherapy, 18*,123–130.

Nucho, A. O. (1987). *The psychocybernetic model of art therapy*. Springfield, IL: Charles C Thomas.

O'Conner, J., & Brown, L. (Eds.). (1978). *Free, adult, uncensored: The living history of the Federal Theater Project*. Washington, DC: New Republic.

Pasto, T. (1962). Meaning in art therapy. *Bulletin of Art Therapy, 2,* 73–76.

Prinzhorn, H. (1972). *Artistry of the mentally ill* (E. von Brockdorff, Trans.). New York, NY: Springer-Verlag. [Originally published in 1922 as *Bildnerei der Geisteskranken.* Berlin: Verlag Julius Springer.]

Rameriz, W. (1971a). Letter in the reader's forum. *American Journal of Art Therapy, 10,* 74.

Rameriz, W. (1971b). Letter in the reader's forum. *American Journal of Art Therapy, 10,* 130.

Rhyne, J. (1973). *The gestalt art experience.* Monterey, CA: Brooks/Cole. [Reprinted in 1984. Chicago, IL: Magnolia Street.]

Rhyne, J. (1975). An oral history: Art therapy pioneers [audio tape]. Louisville, KY: Department of History, University of Louisville.

Rhyne, J. (1987). Gestalt art therapy. In J. A. Rubin (Ed.), *Approaches to art therapy.* New York, NY: Brunner/Mazel.

Robbins, A. (1971). Letter in the reader's forum. *American Journal of Art Therapy, 10,* 99–100.

Robbins, A. (1980). *Expressive therapy: A creative arts approach to depth-oriented treatment.* New York, NY: Human Sciences Press.

Robbins, A. (1987a). *The artist as therapist.* New York, NY: Human Sciences Press.

Robbins, A. (1987b). An object relations approach to art therapy. In J. A. Rubin (Ed.), *Approaches to art therapy.* New York, NY: Brunner/Mazel.

Robbins, A. (1989). *The psychoaesthetic experience.* New York, NY: Human Sciences Press.

Robbins, A. & Sibley, L. B. (1976). *Creative art therapy.* New York, NY: Brunner/Mazel.

Robinson, M. C. (1983). Foreword. *The artist in each of us.* Craftsbury Common, VT: Art Therapy Publications.

Rubin, J. A. (1972). *We'll show you what we're gonna do! (Art for multiply-handicapped blind children),* 16mm. film. New York, NY: ACI Media.

Rubin, J. A. (1973). A diagnostic interview. *Art Psychotherapy, 1,* 31–44.

Rubin, J. A. (1978). *Child art therapy.* New York, NY: Van Nostrand Reinhold.

Rubin, J. A. (1984). *The art of art therapy.* New York, NY: Brunner/Mazel.

Rubin, J. A. (1985). Meet the ole timers: Perspectives on the American Art Therapy Association. Messages in Art. Program of the 16th Annual Conference for the American Art Therapy Association, New Orleans, LA.

Rubin, J. A. (Ed.). (1987a). *Approaches to art therapy.* New York, NY: Brunner/Mazel.

Rubin, J. A. (1987b). Freudian psychoanalytic theory: Emphasis on uncovering and insight. In J. A. Rubin (Ed.), *Approaches to art therapy.* New York, NY: Brunner/Mazel.

Rubin, J. A. (1987c). Conclusion. In J. A. Rubin (Ed.), *Approaches to art therapy.* New York, NY: Brunner/Mazel.

Rubin, J. A. (1994). Personal communication with author (telephone call, January 14).

Sechehaye, M. (1951). *Symbolic realization.* New York, NY: International Universities Press.

Shoemaker, R., Ulman, E., Anderson, F., Wallace, E., Lachman-Chapin, M., Wolf, R., & Kramer, E. (1977). Art therapy: An exploration of definitions. In: R. Shoemaker & S. Gonick-Barris (Eds.), *Creativity and the art therapist's identity,* Proceedings of the 7th Annual AATA Conference. Baltimore, MD: American Art Therapy Association.

Silver, R. A. (1978). *Developing cognitive and creative skills through art.* Baltimore, MD: University Park Press.

Silver, R. A. (1985). Meet the ole timers: Perspectives on the American Art Therapy Association. *Messages in Art*. Program of the 16th Annual Conference for the American Art Therapy Association, New Orleans, LA.

Silver, R. A. (1988). *Draw-a-story: Screening for depression and emotional needs*. Mamaronck, NY: Ablin Press.

Silver, R. A. (1989a). *Developing cognitive and creative skills through art* (3rd ed.) Mamaronck, NY: Ablin Press.

Silver, R.A. (1989b). *Stimulus drawings and techniques: In therapy, development, and assessment* (4th ed. rev.) Mamaronck, NY: Ablin Press.

Silver, R. A. (1990). *Silver drawing test of cognitive skills and adjustment*. Mamaronck, NY: Ablin Press.

Sinrod, H. (1964). Communication through paintings in a therapy group. *Bulletin of Art Therapy, 3,* 133–147.

Slegelis, M. H. (1987). A study of Jung's mandala and its relationship to art psychotherapy. *The Arts in Psychotherapy, 14* , 301–311.

Stern, R. & Honoré, E. (1969). The problem of national organization: Make haste slowly. *Bulletin of Art Therapy, 8,* 91–95.

Stroyman, H. (1971). Letter in the reader's forum. *American Journal of Art Therapy, 10,* 130, 143–144.

Ulman, E. (1960). Psychiatry and the creative process: An exchange of insights. *Psychiatry: Journal for the study of interpersonal processes, 23,* 109–113.

Ulman, E. (1961a). Editorial. *Bulletin of Art Therapy, 1,* 3–5.

Ulman, E. (1961b). Art therapy: Problems of definition. *Bulletin of Art Therapy, 1,* 10–20.

Ulman, E. (1971). Curriculum vitae [unpublished]. Topeka, KS: Archives of the American Art Therapy Association, Menninger Foundation Library.

Ulman, E. (1975a). An oral history: Art therapy pioneers [audio tape]. Louisville, KY: Department of History, University of Louisville.

Ulman, E. (1975b). Art therapy: Problems of defintion. In E. Ulman & P. Dachinger (Eds.), *Art therapy in theory and practice.* New York, NY: Schocken.

Ulman, E. (1975c). Therapy is not enough: The contribution of art to general hospital psychiatry. In E. Ulman & P. Dachinger (Eds.), *Art therapy in theory and practice.* New York, NY: Schocken.

Ulman, E. (1975d). A new use of art in psychiatric diagnosis. In E. Ulman & P. Dachinger (Eds.), *Art therapy in theory and practice.* New York, NY: Schocken.

Ulman, E. (1987). Variations on a Freudian theme: Three art therapy theorists. In J. A. Rubin, (Ed.) *Approaches to art therapy.* New York, NY: Brunner/Mazel.

Ulman, E., Champernowne, I., & members of the staff. (1963). Psychotherapy and the arts at the Withymead Centre, *Bulletin of Art Therapy, 2,* 91–119.

Ulman, E., & Dachinger, P. (Eds.), (1975). *Art therapy in theory and practice.* New York, NY: Schocken.

Ulman, E., Kramer, E., & Kwiatkowska, H. Y. (1978). *Art therapy in the United States.* Craftsbury Common, VT: Art Therapy Publications.

Ulman, E., & Levy, C.A. (Eds.) (1980). *Art therapy viewpoints.* New York, NY: Schocken.

Wadeson, H. (1980). *Art psychotherapy.* New York, NY: John Wiley.

Wadeson, H. (1982). The last lesson. *American Journal of Art Therapy, 21,* 124.

Wadeson, H. (1985). Meet the ole timers: Perspectives on the American Art Therapy Association. Messages in Art. Program of the 16th Annual Conference for the American Art Therapy Association, New Orleans, LA.

Wadeson, H. (1987a). *The dynamics of art psychotherapy*. New York, NY: John Wiley.

Wadeson, H. (1987b). An eclectic approach to art therapy. In J. A. Rubin (Ed.), *Approaches to art therapy*. New York, NY: Brunner/Mazel.

Wadeson, H., Durkin, J., & Perach, D. (Eds.) (1989). *Advances in art therapy*. New York, NY: Wiley.

Wallace, E. (1975). Creativity and Jungian thought. *The Arts in Psychotherapy, 2,* 181–187.

Wallace, E. (1980). Establishing connections between two worlds. In I. Baker (Ed.), *Treatment in analytical psychology*. Felbach: Adolph Borg.

Wallace, E. (1987). Healing through the visual arts — A Jungian approach. In J. A. Rubin (Ed). *Approaches to art therapy*. New York, NY: Brunner/Mazel.

Waller, D. (1992). Different things to different people: Art therapy in Britain—A brief survey of its history and current development. *The Arts in Psychotherapy, 19,* 87–92.

Williams, K. (1992). Obituary: Elinor Ulman (1910–1991). *American Journal of Art Therapy, 30,* 66.

Winnicott, D. (1971). *Playing and reality*. New York, NY: Basic.

Wittels, B. (1982). Interpretations of the "body of water" metaphor in patient artwork as part of the diagnostic process. *The Arts in Psychotherapy, 9,* 177–182.

Wohl, A. & Kaufman, B. (1985). *Silent screams and hidden cries.* New York, NY: Brunner/Mazel.

Yalom, I. (1985). *The theory and practice of group psychotherapy.* New York, NY: Basic.

Zubin, J., Eron, L.D., & Shumer, F. (1965). *A n experimental approach to projective techniques.* New York, NY: John Wiley.

Index

About the Authors

Maxine Borowsky Junge is Associate Professor and Chair of the Marital and Family Therapy Department (Clinical Art Therapy) Loyola Marymount University in Los Angeles. From adolescence, she was trained as a painter at Otis Art Institute, Chouinard Institute, Instituto Allende, Mexico, and did graduate work in painting at U.C.L.A. She holds a Bachelor of Art degree in Art and Humanities from Scripps College, a Master of Social Work from the University of Southern California, and a doctorate in Human and Organizational Systems from the Fielding Institute. Dr. Junge has been an art therapy educator and clinician for more than twenty years. She was formerly a staff member at the National Council of Jewish Women, Thalians Community Mental Health Center - Cedars Sinai Hospital and Ross Loos Medical Group, one of the first health maintenance organizations. She maintains a private practice in Los Angeles. She is the first recipient of an Award for Excellence for her contributions to the development of the art therapy field from the South Bay Contemporary Museum and U.C.L.A./Harbor County Hospital. She is currently completing a book titled *Creative Realities: The Search for Meanings*, a study of visual artists and writers from an alternative realities perspective.

Paige Pateracki Asawa received a Bachelor of Fine Arts from Manhattanville College and taught art to adults for several years which sparked her interest in the healing quality of the art process. She later received a Master of Arts in Marital and Family Therapy (Clinical Art Therapy) from Loyola Marymount University. She graduated with honors as a Helen Landgarten Scholar. She has lectured on her work entitled "Marital imagery: Crossing cultures" at the American Art therapy Association's annual conference and other institutions. Currently, she is in private practice with offices in West Los Angeles and Encino, California. She works with a diverse population including several women's groups and facilitates a series of workshops on recovering and unblocking creativity. She also owns a graphics business, creating layout and design for publications in the fields of music, art therapy, and business including the design for this book.